getting into the
PA SCHOOL
of your choice

Andrew J. Rodican, PA-C

McGraw-Hill
Medical Publishing Division

New York Chicago San Francisco Lisbon London Madrid Mexico City Milan
New Delhi San Juan Seoul Singapore Sydney Toronto

McGraw-Hill

A Division of The **McGraw·Hill** *Companies*

Getting Into the PA School of Your Choice

Copyright © 1998 by Andrew Rodican. All rights reserved. Printed in the United States of America. Except as permitted under the United States Copyright Act of 1976, no part of this publication may be reproduced or distributed in any form or by any means, or stored in a data base or retrieval system, without the prior written permission of the publisher.

2 3 4 5 6 7 8 9 0   CCI/CCI   0 9 8 7 6 5 4 3 2

ISBN: 0-8385-3132-6

Notice

Medicine is an ever-changing science. As new research and clinical experience broaden our knowledge, changes in treatment and drug therapy are required. The authors and the publisher of this work have checked with sources believed to be reliable in their efforts to provide information that is complete and generally in accord with the standards accepted at the time of publication. However, in view of the possibility of human error or changes in medical sciences, neither the authors nor the publisher nor any other party who has been involved in the preparation or publication of this work warrants that the information contained herein is in every respect accurate or complete, and they disclaim all responsibility for any errors or omissions or for the results obtained from use of the information contained in this work. Readers are encouraged to confirm the information contained herein with other sources. For example and in particular, readers are advised to check the product information sheet included in the package of each drug they plan to administer to be certain that the information contained in this work is accurate and that changes have not been made in the recommended dose or in the contraindications for administration. This recommendation is of particular importance in connection with new or infrequently used drugs.

Library of Congress Cataloging-in-Publication Data

Rodican, Andrew J.
    Getting into the PA school of your choice / Andrew J. Rodican.
      p. cm.
    ISBN 0-8385-3132-6 (pbk. : alk. paper)
     1. Physicians' assistants—Education—United States.
2. Physicians' assistants—Vocational guidance. 3. Medical
colleges—United States—Admission. I. Title.
  R697.P45R646 1997
  610.69′53′071173—dc21   97–29065
                                                  CIP

Editor-in-Chief: Cheryl Mehalik
Production Editor: Eileen L. Pendagast
Designer: Janice Barsevich Bielawa

This book is dedicated to the memory of my father,
James A. Rodican

Acknowledgments

I would like to thank my wife, Debbie, for her support, suggestions, and encouragement throughout this entire process. She put up with my absence for too many hours and helped with a great many of the administrative details which went into this project.

I would also like to thank my children, Eddie and Nicole, for their support: Eddie, for his help on the computer which was invaluable, and Nicole, for being so patient.

Finally, I thank my friend, Chuck Ruotolo, for his inspiration and encouragement. Without his idea, this project would not have come to fruition.

A special thanks to my mom, Aurora T. Buckingham ("Nikki"). It was her inspiration as a mother, and a nurse, that influenced my decision to choose a career in health care.

"A special thanks to William Kohlhepp, PA-C"

About the Author

Andrew J. Rodican, PA-C, is a former member of the Yale University School of Medicine, Physician Associate Program Admission's Committee. He has interviewed many PA school applicants, and read and evaluated numerous applications. He is a recipient of the Yale University School of Medicine Physician Associate Program 1994 Medical Writing Award, and he is the writer and developer of the seminar, "Getting Into the PA School of Your Choice." He has an extensive sales background, and won the Dale Carnegie Sales Training Course, Sales Talk Championship and Human Relations Award. He combines his broad knowledge of the admissions process with his sales background to maximize each candidate's potential for acceptance into the PA school of his/her choice.

Contents

Preface

In recent years, a new career path in medicine has opened its doors, that of the physician assistant. The physician assistant is a licensed health professional who works with physician supervision to practice medicine and provide a broad range of diagnostic and therapeutic services. His/her focus is on patient care and may include educational, research, and administrative activities.

The first class of PAs was assembled in the mid-sixties at Duke University and was made up of former navy corpsmen who had a wealth of medical experience, but no area to practice in the civilian world. These initial PAs emerged to fill a need in mostly rural communities as physician extenders.

At the time of this writing, there are 98 accredited and provisionally accredited PA programs. The number of PAs has grown from the first few Duke graduates of the sixties to over 30,000 today. Some areas boast six PA jobs for every graduate. In addition, the US Department of Labor projects a 36 percent increase in PA jobs through the year 2005.

In order to become licensed as a PA in most states, you must graduate from an accredited PA program and pass the national certifying exam administered by the National Commission on Certification of Physician Assistants (NCCPA). At that point, you will receive the designation PA-C. (To date, Mississippi has no licensure system for PAs.)

PAs practice in a variety of areas: Family Practice, Surgery (and specialties), Internal Medicine (and specialties), Emergency Medicine, Occupational Medicine, OB-GYN, Pediatrics, and Psychiatry. PAs perform a variety of duties to include: taking medical histories, performing physical exams, ordering lab tests, diagnosing acute and chronic illnesses, forming treatment plans, counseling patients, educating patients, performing and assisting in surgery, and promoting preventive medicine.

PAs practice in a variety of employment settings to include: solo office, group office, HMOs, hospital in-patient, clinic/hospital out-patient, rural locations, military/veterans' hospitals, and teaching and faculty positions.

PAs can earn from $45,000 to $50,000 to start, to over $100,000 per year depending on the location and nature of the practice. Most PAs are salaried employees, but many also work on salary plus a share of revenue, salary plus bonus, partnerships, or are self-employed.

With the advent of managed care, the future of the PA profession looks bright. However, there are no guarantees and competition for acceptance to a PA program remains keen. Only those best prepared and qualified will gain acceptance. This is the only way that we can be sure our future PAs will carry on the tradition of service and commitment as did the first Duke graduates.

Given that I have been both a PA interviewer and interviewee, I realized the strong need for a forum that could teach applicants how best to prepare an application and interview for PA school. I have found that excellent candidates, with a variety of backgrounds, from all over the country, sometimes floundered when faced with the intricacies of writing an effective narrative statement, or in presenting themselves in the best light to the admissions committee. Consequently, their chances of being interviewed or perhaps accepted to PA school were ruined.

In this book I will share my experiences with you about how I achieved success applying to PA school in my first year. I will show you how to select a program that's right for you and which programs best match your education and experience. Critical areas of the application will be covered, particularly writing the essay/narrative statement, which tends to make or break so many applicants. I will also guide you through the entire interview process, providing you with an inside look behind the scenes of the admissions committee. I will tell you what to expect, when to expect it, and how to handle it. I will cover specific questions that you may be asked, how each question may be interpreted, and what kind of answers the interview panel is looking for.

I have a vast amount of experience with the application and interview process. In addition, I have read hundreds of applications and interviewed numerous applicants over the past several years. In this book you will benefit from these years of experience and gain a competitive edge.

However, this book is not meant to take a poorly qualified applicant and magically turn him or her into a great prospect. Rather, it is meant to help those with the best qualifications, and show them how to polish their skills and perform well on the written application and the interview.

I am confident that if you read this book carefully and apply all of its principles, you will maximize your chances of getting an interview and being accepted to a program of your choice.

Introduction

Congratulations. You are taking the first step toward one of the most important decisions you will probably make in your life. You are embarking on a journey that will take you through two to four years of a rigorous didactic phase, a challenging clinical experience, and a wonderful opportunity to practice medicine as a physician assistant. Along the way, you will pay the price, both financially and emotionally but, in the long run, when you stand up to receive your certificate or your degree, you will know that it has all been worth the struggle.

We have seen many people apply to PA school for many reasons. Some have simply heard about the profession in the newspaper or on TV and thought they would try their luck applying to a program. Others have sought out PAs in clinical practice or know PAs from their work and have spent many hours learning more about the profession. These latter applicants spend their time taking extra classes or volunteering to get more experience. They are like sponges, soaking up every bit of information that they can get on the profession. It is for these people that I write this book.

People may wonder if there really is a need for a book or seminar on getting into PA school. After all, don't you just send in an application and go to the interview, look your best, and smile a lot. If that were the case, we wouldn't have so many excellent candidates being turned down. From reading many applications and interviewing numerous applicants, I've seen highly qualified people, who would surely make very competent PAs, get turned down for making needless mistakes in their applications or in the interview. The competition is such that any tiny error can make the difference between an acceptance letter and a "Thank you anyway."

If you are applying for admission to a physician assistant program, you will quickly find out how competitive this process can be, and you will want answers to these vital questions.

- ▶ Should I apply to a Bachelor's or a Master's program?
- ▶ Why is it so hard to get into PA school?
- ▶ What do I include in the narrative/personal statement?
- ▶ Are all PA schools the same?
- ▶ How do I improve my chances of getting in?
- ▶ What is the interview process like?
- ▶ What does the admissions committee look for in an applicant?

Armed with the answers, you will find a clear pathway ahead on how to accomplish your goal of **getting into the PA school of your choice.**

In addition to reading this book, I highly recommend that you join the American Academy of Physician Assistants (AAPA) as an affiliate member. I also recommend joining your constituent (state) chapter of the AAPA.

List of Contributors

Linda Hricz-Borges, PA-C
George Brothers, PA-S
J.M. Farrell, PA-C
Rosemary Jones
Don Solimini, PA-C
Terry Spahr, PA-C

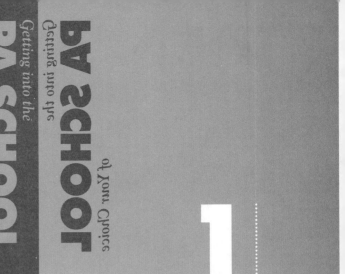

Setting Goals

WHY SET GOALS?

You may be wondering why I add this chapter so early in the book; however, the fact is that so few people ever bother to set goals in life. Most people are what Zig Ziglar calls (in his video, *Goals, Setting and Achieving Them on Schedule*) "a wandering generality," when they need to become "a meaningful specific." The competition for getting into PA school is fierce. Without a written goal and plan of action, your chances of being accepted to the program of your choice are slim.

The basic problem most people have with setting goals is not time, but a lack of direction. Everyone has twenty-four hours in a day. Why is it that some people, who are intelligent and capable, achieve so much, while others, who are equally so, can't seem to get anything accomplished? These people have goals: written, measurable, and realistic. Numerous authors, from Stephen Covey to Norman Vincent Peale, have discussed how to go about goal setting. They agree that specific long- and short-range goals will lead you to become more creative which will, in turn, add more excitement and fulfillment to your life.

Do you know why 97% of people never really set goals in the proper fashion? As Zig Ziglar says, the answer is **FEAR**. False Evidence Appearing Real. Using this principle, you could rob a bank with just your finger in your pocket, or hijack a plane with a fake bomb. But what are we afraid of? There is danger in setting goals. We become afraid that we may not reach them.

However, there is also danger in not setting goals—the danger of wasting our resources.

Did you know that a boat in dry-dock rots quicker than a boat at sea? Don't waste your natural resources; write down your goals today. (See Appendix C.)

If I haven't yet convinced you of the importance of goal setting, perhaps this next story will. In 1953, a study at Yale University polled the graduating seniors with respect to who had written goals and a plan of action for carrying them out. Surprisingly, only three percent of these Ivy Leaguers bothered to take the seven steps necessary to achieve their goals. Only ten percent took some of the steps, and 87% set no goals at all, and had no plan of action for life—"wandering generalities."

> "EVERYONE HAS TALENT. WHAT IS RARE IS THE COURAGE TO FOLLOW THE TALENT TO THE DARK PLACE WHERE IT LEADS."
>
> *Erica Jong, The Passionate State of Mind.*

> "FEAR IS A NOOSE THAT BINDS UNTIL IT STRANGLES."
>
> *Jean Toomer, Definitions and Aphorisms, XVI, 1931.*

In 1973, those same graduating seniors were re-polled in areas which were considered measurable: finances, career, position in life. Not surprisingly, those three percent of people who had set goals, and followed a plan of action to carry them out, accomplished more than the other 97% combined.

SEVEN-STEP FORMULA FOR SUCCESS

If you know this seven-step formula for success, it won't make a difference what the goal is, you'll be able to accomplish it. By knowing and following these seven steps you will maximize your chances of getting into the PA school of your choice.

1. Identify the goal
2. Set a deadline for achievement
3. List obstacles to overcome
4. Identify people and organizations who can help you
5. List the skills and knowledge required to achieve your goal
6. Develop a plan of action
7. List the benefits of achieving the goal; ask yourself, "What's in it for me?"

Now what I would like you to do is to take out your pencil and paper and begin listing your goals. If you do nothing else with this book, I'll consider this one action step a success if you complete your goal sheet. If you need some help getting started, let's look at an example of my written goal for getting into PA school in 1992. (You will notice that I wrote my goal in paragraph form. You can write your goals however you prefer.)

August 15, 1990

By May 1, 1992 I will be accepted into either Yale, the University of Florida, or Bowman Gray's Physician Assistant Program. In order to accomplish this goal, I will first have to discuss my desire to become a PA with my wife and convince her that this is the right thing to do for our family. Next, I will need to begin saving money so that I can help my wife support our two children and provide food and shelter for two years. Finally, I will stay focused and not listen to those people who will say I'm "crazy" or having an "early mid-life crisis" for wanting to quit a great job at age 35 and go back to school for two years.

I will immediately contact the AAPA and ConnAPA to find out what resources are available to me. I will get a PA program directory and begin writing to several PA schools, focusing on my top three. I will contact the president of ConnAPA and get to know him. I will also visit Yale's PA program and visit with Elaine Grant, who is the Dean of the program, and maintain contact with her quarterly. I will do the same thing at the other two programs. I will find out from these people what I lack as a competitive candidate and how I can best strengthen my application.

I will visit with some PAs who work in my wife's office and spend as much time with them as possible. I will attend as many open houses as possible to learn more about each program and to make myself known to them.

I will need Anatomy and Physiology (I & II) and Microbiology to fulfill requirements. I will achieve no less than an A in each class. I will also begin volunteering at Saint Raphael's hospital, in the ER, in order to gain more "recent" experience. I will also obtain an SAT study guide to prepare myself for the test, which I need to take to get into Yale.

My plan is to continue working full time, save the money I need, and volunteer part time. I will also take evening classes. While working in the hospital, I will discuss my goals with as many PAs as possible and learn as much as I can about the PA profession.

Once I achieve my goal of getting into the PA school of my choice, I will enjoy many benefits: helping people, job satisfaction, secure future, challenging work, stimulating work, prestige, a sense of accomplishment, and much more.

I wrote these goals in 1990. I can also vividly remember the exact moment that I decided to apply to PA school. I was on vacation with my wife and children in Florida. I was in my friend Chuck's office looking through the classifieds when I spotted a job for a Plastic Surgery PA. On a whim, I called the number and spoke to the office secretary. She practically begged me to come in for an interview. In my excitement I forgot to tell her that I wasn't a PA at all, but I didn't want to ruin a nice conversation. It was at that moment that I told Chuck I was going to apply to PA school. He said, "Go for it!" and I haven't looked back since.

Here's another example of someone who, having put a hurried application together for PA school and failed to get in, re-assessed his priorities and concentrated on new goals.

I planned for things to be different next year. I would:

▶ identify schools I could apply to using the APAP directory of PA programs
▶ apply to at least five new schools to increase the opportunity of being interviewed
▶ request and complete a school's application as soon as it was available
▶ type and proofread everything I sent to the program
▶ join the AAPA as an affiliate member
▶ visit as many programs as I could during a summer trip east
▶ continue to take classes that would prepare me for PA school

By the end of the year I had applied to nine schools. I had attended one interview and had three more after the first of the year. To prepare for these, I read several interview books and bought a new suit. I studied up on some of the issues facing the profession and health care in general. I tried to relax. The interviews were similar in format, as were the questions. Then I had to wait. Two weeks after the last interview, I was notified by the school that was my top choice that I was accepted. The years of going to school during the day and working at night, the preparation for interviews, and the tiring trips across the country had all paid off. I was in.

George Brothers

This brings me to another topic that I would like to discuss with you; it's called "imaging." It's a technique that I learned in Officer's Training School (USAF), and it's a powerful tool. You may have heard the saying "What the mind can conceive and believe it can achieve." Nothing could be more true. Get used to seeing yourself opening that acceptance letter, or performing well at the interview. Every day spend some time meditating on your goal. You'll be surprised at the results you'll get. I used to work out on my Nordictrack every day for a half-hour and visualize myself getting the acceptance letter. That's over 180 hours of imaging; it's powerful and it works.

My efforts paid off. I interviewed at the University of Florida in December 1991 on a Friday. The next Monday they called to tell me that I was accepted. I also got accepted into Yale's program in March 1992. I chose to stay local and go to Yale, so I did not have to fly to North Carolina and interview at Bowman Gray. I had achieved my goal of getting into the PA school of my choice by having a written goal, working hard, and simply carrying out a plan of action.

TAKE A PERSONAL EVALUATION

Periodically, you must review your performance and evaluate which areas you need improvement in. There are seven specific areas to look at:

1. Appearance
2. Family
3. Financial
4. Social
5. Spiritual
6. Mental
7. Career

Every so often take a look at these areas and ask yourself questions like:

► Do I present myself well? Do I need to lose some weight or buy some new shoes?
► Is my family behind me? Will this career change cause tension in my marriage or relationship? Am I willing to listen to the skeptics?
► Can I afford to go to school now? Does the school offer graduate level loans? Can I save enough money between now and the time school starts?
► Am I a team player? Will I be able to work as a "dependent" practitioner? Do I get along well with people?
► Is it morally right for me to do this now? Do I have other obligations or responsibilities? Am I being selfish?
► Should I retake any courses? Am I well read on medical issues and current events? Will I be able to concentrate on my course work?
► Do I really know why I want to be a PA? Am I sure I want to do this? Do I really know what PAs do?

Score your answers in these seven areas on a scale from 1 to 5, with five being the highest and one being the lowest. Work on those areas in which you score low. Doing this periodically will keep you on course and help you reach your goals quicker.

SET BIG GOALS

There were once two men fishing on a pier; one old and one young. The young man watched as the older man kept reeling in big fish but throwing them back into the water. "Why are you throwing back those big, beautiful fish?" asked the young man. "Because I only have this little frying pan," said the old man, holding up a scrawny little skillet. (Zig Ziglar)

Set big goals and **go for the gold!** Dig down deep into your soul and focus on what you want in life. Make a plan and see yourself accomplishing it. Emerson once wrote, "What lies behind us and what lies in front of us, pales in significance to what lies within us."

WHO DO I SHARE MY GOALS WITH

The rule here is that you share "give up" goals with everybody, and "go up" goals with the people you love and trust. For example, if you want to lose twenty pounds, let everybody at home and at the office know about it; this is a "give up" goal. But if you want to get into PA school, tell only your family and close friends. They will give you an honest opinion and support you, while others may offer negativity and skepticism.

To keep yourself focused, write this down on your mirror, or a place where you'll see it often each day:

> Obstacles are those frightful things you see when you take your eyes off your goal.
>
> *Henry Ford*

Each time you have a sinking feeling in the pit of your stomach, and you start to think that you may have bitten off more than you can chew, take a look at the above statement. Know that you can do anything you set your mind to as long as you stay focused.

MAKE A COMMITMENT

In closing this chapter, I would like to encourage you to make a commitment to your goal, yourself, your family, and your life. Be positive, use daily vocabulary like, "I will . . . , I can . . . , When I get into PA school . . . " Avoid negative thinking like, "If I do . . . , If I can . . . , If I get into PA school . . . " Remember, you don't pay the price for setting goals, you enjoy the benefits of reaching them.

YOU DON'T PAY THE PRICE FOR SETTING GOALS, YOU ENJOY THE BENEFITS OF REACHING THEM.

Selecting a Program

2

You may be asking at this point, aren't all programs the same? What difference does it make which program I attend as long as I will become a PA? These are good questions, and, for the most part, you may be right. However, there are several issues that you need to consider prior to applying to a PA program. Why spend a great deal of energy and money applying to a particular school only to find out later that you can't really afford it or that they prefer students from their home state. This chapter will open your eyes to some of the things you must look for when applying to any program.

At this time we would like to encourage you, once again, to join the American Academy of Physician Assistants (AAPA) as an affiliate member, and your state chapter of the AAPA as an affiliate member. To join the AAPA call or write:

> The American Academy of Physician Assistants
> 950 N. Washington Street
> Alexandria, VA 22314-1552
> (703) 836-2272

To join your state chapter, see Appendix D.

> The American Academy of
> Physician Assistants
> 950 N. Washington Street
> Alexandria, VA 22314-1552
> (703) 836-2272

ACCREDITATION

First and foremost, you want to make sure that the program you are attending is accredited by the Commission on Accreditation of Allied Health Education Programs (CAAHEP). The Accreditation Review Committee on Education for the Physician Assistant (ARC-PA) includes representatives from the American Medical Association (AMA), the Association of Physician Assistant Programs (APAP), the American Academy of Family Physicians, the American Academy of Pediatrics, the American College of Physicians, and the American College of Surgeons. As of this writing, there are 98 accredited PA programs.

If you do not graduate from an accredited program, you will not be eligible to take the national certifying examination for physician assistants which is administered by the National Commission on Certification of Physician Assistants (NCCPA). Without your NCCPA license, you will not be able to practice medicine in most locations.

If you are applying to a brand new program, ask if they have applied for provisional accreditation. This means that they will have received a comprehensive evaluation prior to opening. Although having this evaluation does not guarantee accreditation, at least you can get an idea of where the program stands in the process.

If you have any questions regarding accreditation issues, contact:

Accreditation Review Committee on Education for the
    Physician Assistant
1000 North Oak Avenue
Marshfield, WI 54449-5788
(715) 389-3785

Accreditation Review
    Committee on Education for
    the Physician Assistant
1000 North Oak Avenue
Marshfield, WI 54449-5788
(715) 389-3785

FOCUS OF THE PROGRAM

Mostly all admissions committees select applicants based on several factors that include, but are not limited to: academics, test scores (SAT, GRE, AHPAT, TOEFL, etc.), understanding of the PA concept, health care experience, volunteer work, community service, interviews, the narrative statement, and references. Certain programs, however, do mention in their selection criteria what the focus of their program may be, or which type of student they prefer. By knowing this ahead of time you can concentrate your energies on a program that best suits your needs.

The following list will give you an idea about which programs specifically mention **key words** in their "selection factor" section of their brochures. These are not always absolute criteria, and you should contact each program for further information.

PRACTICE IN MEDICALLY UNDER-SERVED AREAS

Charles R. Drew University of Medicine and Science
University at California, Davis
Stanford University
University of Southern California School of Medicine—"recruiting disadvantaged applicants"
George Washington University—"recruiting disadvantaged applicants"
Emory University School of Medicine
Augsburg College
City University of New York/ Harlem Hospital Center
University of North Dakota School of Medicine
Oregon Health Sciences University
Philadelphia College of Textiles and Science
University of Utah School of Medicine

STATE RESIDENTS RECEIVE PREFERENCE

Charles R. Drew University of Medicine and Science
Medical College of Georgia
Cook County Hospital/ Malcolm X College
Wichita State University
University of South Dakota (tri-state: NE Nebraska, NW Iowa, and SE South Dakota)

Oregon Health Sciences University
Bowman Gray School of Medicine of Wake Forest
The University of Texas Medical Branch
University of Utah School of Medicine (intermountain west region)

PRIMARY CARE

Emory University School of Medicine
Albany-Hudson
Bayley-Seton Hospital
Oregon Health Sciences University

SURGEON ASSISTANT PROGRAMS

University of Alabama at Birmingham
Cornell University Medical College
Cuyahoga Community College

NURSING BACKGROUND

University of North Dakota School of Medicine

PHYSICIAN PRECEPTOR

University of California, Davis

TEST SCORES

University of Colorado School of Medicine
King's College
Medical College of Pennsylvania and Hahnemann University

WELL-DEFINED GOALS

Touro College of Health Sciences
Kettering College of Medical Arts

CHRISTIAN SERVICE

Trevecca Nazarene University

FLUENCY IN SPANISH

The University of Texas Medical Branch

Do not become intimidated by the above list. I personally know of several George Washington University students who are neither "disadvantaged" nor working in "under-served" areas. I recently interviewed a graduate of North Dakota's program for a cardiothoracic surgery job. There are plenty of exceptions to every program listed above. No program can force you to work in that state after you graduate. There is nothing to stop a graduate from a "surgeon assistant" program from working in primary care. The point to listing these preferences is to key you in on what the admissions committee may be looking for when they see your application, or when they interview you.

THE EDUCATIONAL EXPERIENCE

Before we get to the issue of Master's versus Bachelor's, let's look at the degrees and certificates some of the programs have to offer and discuss the issues that may be important to you when selecting your program.

First of all, there are Master's programs, graduate programs, and undergraduate programs. In some of these schools you'll receive a degree, and in others a certificate. As long as your school is accredited, and you become certified, you can work as a PA. But everyone is looking for different challenges in a program. Some programs have a cadaver lab for anatomy and physiology; others use slides or models. Some programs are taught by residents, fellows, and attending physicians; others use a self-taught, small group learning approach. Some programs are affiliated with a medical school, with all the benefits of that facility. Others are located at community colleges. In addition, as the saying goes, "you get what you pay for," and when you look at the costs of some of these programs (see financial aid section) you will see a great diversity in price. Only you know what you can afford or what you are willing to invest for your education.

MASTER'S VERSUS BACHELOR'S

One of the most frequently asked questions is: "Does it matter if you have a Master's or a Bachelor's degree?" The answer is: "No," if you want to practice medicine, and "Maybe," if you want to teach or get into administration. Even then you can always get a Master's later, and perhaps, at your employer's expense. With all of the people we interview at our hospital we never even ask them if they have a Master's degree. We just want to know if they're certified, and, in our cardiac surgery department, if they can tie a knot, or put in a chest tube. In this age of six jobs for every graduate, whether you have a Master's will not necessarily give you the edge over anyone else. Employers just want PAs.

On the other hand, if your program offers a Master's option, or if you get accepted to both a Master's and a Bachelor's program, for example, then you may have to give the matter additional thought. But keep in mind that, as mentioned already, "you get what you pay for," and it will cost you more for that extra piece of paper which you will not recoup on the job, at least initially. However, if you have in mind a teaching or faculty position in the future, then a Master's is what you will need.

PASS/FAIL RATE

Even more important than which degree or certificate a program offers is the first-time pass/fail rate. If only 50% of the graduates pass their national board exam the first time around, then the significance of a Master's course may not seem so paramount. Be sure to specify "first-time" when you inquire about this very important number. Some programs may just give you an overall pass/fail rate, meaning eventually 90%, or 80% pass the boards. You should know that once you've already failed, your odds of passing the boards decrease significantly each time you take the exam. Part of the reason for this is that if you fail, you can't work, and you have to wait six months to take the exam again. That means no clinical experience, and some say this is where you gain most of your knowledge for board questions—working with actual patients.

OTHER ISSUES TO CONSIDER

We have already covered some of the main points to think about when selecting a program; now we will look at some other issues which may influence your decision.

CLINICAL ROTATIONS

Once you complete your didactic training, you will go out on rotations and practice your clinical skills. You will collect and perform histories and physical examinations (H&Ps) on actual patients and you will have to learn the intricacies of each facility you work in. You will find that just as you become comfortable at the rotation site, and you've learned where the bathroom and cafeteria are, it's time to move on.

You should become familiar with the rotation selection process before you decide on a school. Most schools have mandatory rotations: OB-GYN, emergency medicine, pediatrics, surgery, medicine, psychiatry, family practice, as well as a wide variety of elective rotations. It is important to find out what the school you are applying to offers. You are the one paying for the education.

Also, find out at what point you will know when and where your rotations will be. Usually, students can pick their rotations and sites on a "dream sheet" several months before entering the clinical phase. You may not get all of the sites that you ask for, but at least you know well in advance exactly where you're going and when you'll be there. This is especially important for those of you who work part-time or have families.

Another good idea is to talk to current students in the program and see how they are enjoying their experience on clinical rotations. Ask them about the ratio of PA students to medical students; are PAs given adequate access to the training experience or do medical students take preference? Most places will offer several rotation sites per each individual rotation. Some of the newer programs may not be as well established at certain sites. You may have to be very assertive to get the educational experience you deserve.

Some programs will keep a running file, compiled by their students, in which the students write an evaluation of each particular rotation and rotation site. They will point out the advantages and disadvantages of the rotation and tell you about parking and housing and other important details.

PARKING AND HOUSING

How will you get to class every day? Can you afford to live in the town where you are going to school? You must consider these issues before you decide on going to any given program. Take into account the cost of living, parking, and housing. A good place to start is the local Chamber of Commerce. They will be glad to send you plenty of information for the asking.

MORE TIPS

The following is a short list of tips to help you select a program. If you follow these suggestions, you will be well informed when it's time to apply and interview.

ORDER THE PA PROGRAMS DIRECTORY

This directory is published each year and is distributed in February. It is a useful guide to each of the PA programs offered in the country and outlines each program's characteristics.

ATTEND THE OPEN HOUSE

This is a must if you're serious about the program. First of all, it gives the program an opportunity to place your face with your name. Most programs

ASK EACH PROGRAM ABOUT THEIR CLINICAL ROTATION SCHEDULE, INCLUDING MANDATORY AND ELECTIVE ROTATIONS.

COMMUNICATE WITH AS MANY STUDENTS AS YOU CAN. THE STUDENT ACADEMY OF THE AAPA (SAAAPA) WEB SITE IS LOCATED AT:

www.aapa.org/saaapa/

THE PA PROGRAMS DIRECTORY IS A "MUST HAVE" FOR THE SERIOUS APPLICANT. TO ORDER CALL:

1-800-708-7581

will also keep track of who comes to the open house, which may score you a couple of extra points on your application (if you mention it) or at the interview.

Second, you will get a better insight into the philosophy of the program by listening to the guest speakers and being able to talk with the students. **You may even chat with someone who'll be interviewing you later.** Of course, going to the open house doesn't guarantee you an interview, but in this highly competitive environment it doesn't hurt either.

Next, you will have an opportunity to talk with the other applicants and get to "size up" the competition, if you will. Maybe you will get some ideas on how you can strengthen your application. Take this opportunity to soak up as much information as you can from everyone you meet.

Finally, after attending the open house, you may decide on not going or applying to that program. Perhaps you are not impressed with the faculty or the students and you can't see yourself going there. It will be good to find that out sooner rather than later, when you may have already been accepted.

SPEAK WITH THE PROGRAM DIRECTOR

Whether you attend the open house or not, you should call the school of your choice and ask to speak with the Program Director. If you live nearby or plan on visiting, set up an appointment and speak to her or him in person. Again, this gives you a chance to let the program get to know you and place your name with your face. If you do this, however, make sure you dress appropriately and present yourself as you would for an interview. Also, ask appropriate questions (more on this later).

VISIT LOCAL HOSPITALS OR CLINICS

Stop by the local hospital or clinic and see how many of the program's graduates are working there. Ask the physicians and nurses how they feel about PAs and what they think of the local PA program. If you get a favorable response and there are plenty of PAs working in the area, then great. But, if the response is cool or you don't see any of the local graduates at work, perhaps you had better find out why.

THE INTERNET

If you want to communicate with students of any given program, there is a wonderful new web site called "National PA Student Homepage." This page is a great reference and allows you to contact PA students from just about any program in the country by going to the "National PA Student Directory." The site's address is:

http://members.aol.com/medicjer/

Another good idea is to join the PA Forum on the internet. This is a forum in which PAs, PA students, PA faculty, and anyone interested in the PA profession can communicate about issues facing the profession and our community as a whole. This is a great place to learn about current topics in the news: managed care, health care reform, Medicare and Medicaid, etc. The subscription is free. To join:

Prepare e-mail message for: Majordomo@list.mc.duke.edu

Type in **body** of message: subscribe paforum

Or: subscribe studentpa

Once you have completed the above two steps, you will be sent back a message welcoming you to the forum. You should respond with your name and tell a little about yourself. To e-mail the forum, type:

paforum@list.mc.duke.edu

You can subscribe to any other PA forum by typing: subscribe pajournal, subscribe studentpa, subscribe pafaculty, subscribe primarypa.

E-mail the AAPA at:
aapa@aapa.org

interview because of a spelling error or a poorly written letter of reference. You can only hope that you made the correct choices and wonder if, perhaps, the few that came close will interview and be accepted elsewhere.

LETTERS OF RECOMMENDATION

As part of the application process, you will be required to provide at least three letters of recommendation, usually from a PA, a supervisor, and a personal acquaintance or physician. Again, please be sure to pay attention to detail when reading the application package and provide exactly what the program asks for.

When you think about potential references **be sure to include at least one PA.** After all, you are applying to a physician assistant program. This may seem quite obvious to you, but believe me, plenty of people ignore this critical rule. Applicants will mention in their narrative statements that they have worked with PAs and shadowed PAs, but they don't have a PA reference. Make the most of the resources you have available.

Most of these people are under the impression that the bigger the name or position, the better the reference. Nothing could be further from the truth. The admissions committee is made up mostly of PAs. We want to see what our fellow PAs think about you. If you don't know a PA, perhaps you should reconsider your career choice. Otherwise, get busy shadowing a PA or meeting PAs and discussing your plans. Most of us enjoy talking about our profession and would be glad to have you shadow us at work.

Your references will usually be asked to rate you in the following areas:

- ▶ Academic performance
- ▶ Interpersonal skills
- ▶ Maturity
- ▶ Adaptability/flexibility
- ▶ Motivation for a career as a PA

In addition, they will ask for written comments on the following:

- ▶ Applicant's ability to relate well with others
- ▶ Strengths relative to a career as a PA
- ▶ Weaknesses
- ▶ Other comments bearing on the individual applicant

Keep in mind that a good letter of recommendation has four important features:

1. It shows that the writer truly knows the individual and can comment about the applicant's qualifications.
2. It shows that the writer knows enough about the applicant and can make comparative judgments about the applicant's intellectual, academic, and professional abilities in relation to others in a similar role.
3. It provides supporting details to make the statement believable.
4. It is short, yet concise and sincere.

Perhaps we can learn a lesson from our military friends. Both enlisted and officer personnel write their own evaluations for promotion and simply present them to their superiors for signature. This is a common practice. If the supervisor doesn't agree he/she can change it, but that usually doesn't hap-

RATHER THAN USING THE "BIG SHOT" MD FOR A REFERENCE, USE PEOPLE WHO KNOW YOU AND CAN COMMENT ON SPECIFIC ACHIEVEMENTS.

Four Important Features of a Good Letter of Recommendation

pen. If you're concerned that the person you're using as a reference is too busy, or maybe doesn't have the best writing skills, you write the reference and have him or her sign it. There is nothing wrong with this as long as you don't forget any signatures. (See Appendix B.)

Finally, **follow up** on your letters of reference. If your writer needs to be reminded to submit your letter, do it tactfully, but assertively. This is your future at stake here. This is another reason to avoid the "big names" when obtaining references. It can be difficult to get in touch with them, or they may be too busy to write an effective letter of reference.

In summary, the letter of reference plays a vital role in the evaluation of your application. **The key to this part of the process is to use a PA.** If you absolutely can't obtain a PA reference, ask someone who knows you well and can honestly, and enthusiastically, comment on your desire and ability to be a good PA.

UNIVERSAL RECOMMENDATION LETTER

The Universal Recommendation is an optional letter of recommendation form that you may use in place of individual schools' recommendation forms when you apply to more than one of the participating PA programs.

This service makes it easier to apply to as many programs as you like because your evaluators will only need to fill out one recommendation form instead of a separate one for each school to which you apply. In addition, by using the Universal Letter of Recommendation form you are assured that the quality of your evaluation will not deteriorate as the evaluator fills out multiple forms.

To find out more information on this service, call or write to:

Autumn Jennings
Universal Recommendations
PO Box 18700
Salt Lake City, UT 84118-0700
(801) 969-6085
www.applicants.com

The Narrative Statement

Before you begin to think about writing your narrative statement (essay), take the time to fill out the worksheets at the end of this chapter. We've included several sheets so that you can gather data on your work history, medical experience, high school and college work, volunteer activities, military experience, foreign language abilities, travel experiences, and miscellaneous items. By filling out these forms before you start to write your essay, you will have organized your thoughts so that you can write a more effective essay and, in addition, perform better in your interview.

THE ESSAY IS YOUR TICKET TO THE INTERVIEW.

HOW IMPORTANT IS THE NARRATIVE STATEMENT?

If you were to poll 100 admissions committee members, over 90% would probably tell you that the narrative statement is the **most important** part of the application. This is one of the only parts of the application process that you have any control over. Yes, grade point average, test scores, medical experience, and letters of recommendation are also very important. However, if you fail to connect with the reader of your application on an emotional level, via your narrative, you may be passed over for an interview. In fact, otherwise average candidates receive interviews strictly based on a very effective, emotionally charged essay.

The serious candidate spends a considerable amount of time writing and rewriting the narrative statement. She has several people read the essay for flow, content, grammar, typos, and spelling. A good idea is to read your essay backwards. This is also a great way to catch spelling errors and typos.

The following suggestions will help you to write an effective narrative statement. Do not become frustrated if you have trouble finding the exact words at first. The key is to put the pen to the paper and, as a famous sneaker company suggests, "just do it." **Under no circumstances should you allow someone else to write your essay.** This can be a fatal mistake.

SUGGESTIONS

1. Learn About the Program You're Applying to

If you are going to spend the time, money, and effort applying to a PA program, at least attempt to learn everything that you can about the schools you are applying to. The serious candidate studies the history of the program (and the university or college), the philosophy of the program, and the goals the program sets for educating PA students. Contact as many students and graduates of the program you are applying to, and get a good feel for the strong points and the weak points of the program. Do your homework: it will pay off.

2. Follow Instructions

Carefully read the essay question(s) and answer it (them). Too many of us have our own agenda; we want to tell the readers of our essay what *we* want them to hear, rather than what they are asking us for. For example, if you are asked "How do you expect to fulfill your goals as a physician assistant?," don't write about your prior experiences saving lives and volunteering in the soup kitchen; answer the question!

In addition, if they ask for a two-page narrative, don't write three pages. In this case more is not better. Imagine a committee member reading her 100th application and she comes across a "three pager," with size 8 font. Don't give the reader any excuse for not giving your essay the attention it deserves.

3. Avoid Using "I" Too Much

Nothing is worse than someone focusing on their achievements and saying "I did this . . ." and then "I did that . . ." Use "we," "us," and "our" more often. Give the reader the impression that you are a team player. Talk more about your patients. At one open house I attended, we were told that if we had more than five "I's" in our essay we should do it over. Now this may be stretching it a bit, but I'm sure a lot of essays got re-worked after that open house ended.

4. Target Your Audience

Remember that most committee members are PAs. Don't waste precious space in your essay writing about the functions and role of the PA. Believe it or not, many people waste up to a half page repeating the AAPA definition of a physician assistant. Use this space to tell the reader what separates you from the other ten candidates hoping to get your interview slot.

5. Make It Presentable

It goes without saying that you should type your essay on a computer and have it laser printed. If you are instructed to do otherwise, then **follow instructions.** Do not type in small fonts; use size 12.

6. Check for Spelling

Spelling errors are **inexcusable** and show a complete lack of attention to detail. The message you are sending to the committee is that you don't care enough about your application, and their program, to give your best effort. This is a sure way to be rejected for an interview. Once you finish your essay, run it through a spell checker, then have someone you trust read it and provide you with feedback.

7. Organize Your Writing

Communicating effectively is a key part of the PA's role. If your thoughts are scattered, and you cannot get organized, you will have a great deal of difficulty when it comes to explaining procedures to your patients or presenting a patient's symptoms to your attending physician on rounds.

Programs will often ask you to answer one or more questions in your essay. One program asks you to answer the following: "Attach to this application a **typewritten** narrative of **not more than two pages,** explaining where you learned of the PA profession, what factors or influences led you to this career choice, and how you expect to fulfill your goals as a physician associate." Other programs will simply ask you to explain why you want to become a physician assistant. Still other programs may leave the topic up to you (more about this in the next section). Whichever situation applies to you, be sure to read the question carefully and follow directions.

TOPICS: SELECTION AND DEVELOPMENT

If you have an open-ended essay question, consider one of these to write about:

1. Your motivation for a career as a physician assistant.
2. The influences of your family/early experiences on your life.
3. The influence of extracurricular or work/volunteer activities on your life.
4. Your long-term goals.
5. Your personal philosophy.

GUIDELINES

1. Select only those for which you have something meaningful to say.
2. Convey your personality in your essay; make yourself appear as an interesting candidate to meet and interview.
3. Add "life" to your essay. What's important to you? What experiences impacted on your life? What did you learn as a result of your experiences?
4. Avoid using contractions in an essay. For example, use "did not" versus "didn't" and "I am" versus "I'm."
5. Avoid using abbreviations in your essay unless you have used the complete term first. For example, physician assistant (PA) and emergency room (ER). In general, keep your essay more formal and avoid using abbreviations as much as possible.
6. Avoid slang or colloquial expressions. For example, instead of saying, "He is a really cool professor . . ." use, " He is a good role model . . ."
7. Avoid using run-on sentences. In other words, **keep it simple** by avoiding long sentences with excessive punctuation marks.
8. Make sure your opening paragraph is strong, well constructed, and quickly gains the attention of the reader.
9. Have a key sentence or topic sentence in each paragraph which highlights the main point of the paragraph.
10. Use vignettes, or small anecdotes as examples to back up what you say. Balance these with explanation.
11. Check the use of tenses and make sure they are consistent.
12. Avoid the use of the passive voice; it can be awkward and less effective than the active voice. For example, instead of using "The

job could not be kept because . . .," try "I could not keep the job because . . ."

13. Avoid being too wordy.
14. Conclude your essay as strongly as you began it, with a reiteration of why you want to be a PA (or what your goals are, etc.). A reiteration can add a slightly different slant to what you have already said.

MOTIVATION FOR BECOMING A PA

You should write about your motivation for a career as a physician assistant. I guarantee you that at some point during the interview they'll ask you why you want to become a PA. If you discuss this in the essay, you can deal with this question before it is asked and have a helpful outline to work with.

The first thing to do is spend some quiet time thinking about why you want to become a PA. Do some brainstorming. What experiences or people have led you to this career path? Use examples and vignettes to illustrate your point and lend credibility to your essay. The following example illustrates the point:

> Although there were several excellent doctors in our pediatricians' office, we preferred using the physician assistants on our visits. The pediatricians seemed always rushed and spent little time with the physical exam; they were almost mechanical in their mannerisms. The PAs spent much more time with us and developed a special relationship with our children. They knew what sports my children were involved in, what grades they received in school, and had an overall sense of their well being. Each visit the PA would allow the children to listen to their own heartbeats, and always explained every single procedure before she performed it. I later shadowed this same PA and found out that she grew up with a lot of hardship living in a rural southern community. Yet, she had a tremendous following of patients and enjoyed every minute of her job. I believe a career as a physician assistant can give me the same satisfaction. Becoming a physician assistant will allow me to work autonomously, yet collaboratively, with several members of the health care team. I'll look forward to the first time I get to hold a stethoscope up to a child's heart and ask, "Can you hear it?"

Take out a fresh sheet of paper and write this question at the top, **Why do I want to become a physician assistant?**

Start brainstorming and writing down everything that comes to mind; everything goes. If you find that you are having a hard time coming up with the answers, then answer the questions below to try and focus your thoughts.

Why don't I want to become a physician?

Why don't I want to become a nurse?

Why don't I want to become a nurse practitioner?

Why don't I want to become a teacher?

Why don't I want to become a physical therapist?

Hopefully, you will now have a better understanding of why you want to become a PA. If you are still having difficulty coming up with answers, perhaps you should think hard about choosing this career path.

FAMILY BACKGROUND

Many applicants feel that they must write about medical experiences or educational awards to show that they have value. By writing about individuals or incidents which have shaped your life, you begin to paint a picture of an interesting person, someone the admissions committee would like to meet.

PAINT A PICTURE OF AN INTERESTING PERSON TO MEET AND INTERVIEW.

I grew up one of six children. My father died when I was seven, and my mom worked two jobs to support us. She, fortunately, had an education behind her and worked as a nurse in an emergency room. I grew up with plenty of food on the table and a roof over my head, but I had very little guidance. I often got into trouble and felt lost in life. I did play a lot of sports, though, and, as a result, spent numerous hours in the emergency room where my mom worked. It was here that I became fascinated with medicine. I would peek around corners to watch the doctors perform procedures on patients, and beg my mother to let me stay longer. I felt exhilarated in this environment. One day I shared my feelings with one of the residents. He made a statement which I have not forgotten to this day. He said, "Son, you can become anything you want to in life, if you only set your mind to it."

As I grew older, still with no real direction in life, I often thought about those words but never totally bought into the idea. I quit high school at age sixteen with plans to join the Navy at seventeen. My mother quickly intervened, however, and arranged for me to finish high school during the summer.

That summer, soon after graduation, I enlisted in the Navy and became a hospital corpsman. I grew up and matured a great deal in this environment. Most of all, however, I realized why I had such a fascination for medicine. I loved working in the collaborative environment with other health care professionals. I enjoyed providing care to my fellow servicemen and the satisfaction I felt after sewing a Marine's leg wound in the field or diagnosing an acute appendix in the clinic. For the first time in my life, I actually enjoyed waking up and going to work in the morning. I looked forward to the challenges that lay ahead. I became eager to learn all that I could and began taking college science courses in the evening. I did very well and began to believe that I could do anything that I set my mind to.

As a result of these experiences, I feel that I have a good understanding of what it takes to provide health care. I understand the role of the physician assistant, and I would like to continue my health care experience and aspirations in this newly expanded role.

EXTRACURRICULAR ACTIVITIES AND WORK/VOLUNTEER EXPERIENCES

If you have filled out the worksheets that we provide for you, this should be an easy topic on which to write. Keep in mind that you don't always have to write about medical experiences. Show the reader what you have learned from all of your life experiences and try to demonstrate, in your writing, that you are a person of value. Don't simply repeat items (awards, honors, etc.) that you have listed on the application and is readily available to the reader.

To help you write effectively, think about answering the following questions in your writing:

1. What did you learn from your extracurricular activities or work experiences?
2. Are you a team player?

3. How have you matured as a result of your experiences?
4. If you had a leadership role, how did you contribute to getting the job done?

The key to success in this area is to lead the reader to believe, on his/her own, that you are an independent thinker and a mature person, without actually using these adjectives in your essay.

The following paragraphs, from two essays, illustrate the point I am trying to make. These writers share what they learned from volunteer and work experiences.

CONVINCE THE READER THAT YOU ARE AN INDEPENDENT THINKER AND A MATURE PERSON.

SAMPLE A

When I decided to volunteer at Saint Vincent's hospital, I felt that I had a fairly good idea of how things worked in an emergency room. After all, I worked as an emergency room technician in one of the largest hospitals in the country. What I did not know, however, was how impersonal and insensitive we can be to our patients. In my role as a patient representative I now viewed things from the other side of the fence: the patient's side. I soon realized that the staff frequently referred to the patient as the "leg" in room two, or the "belly" in room five. We tell patients , "Your LFTs are elevated" but never stop to explain what "LFTs" are. We sometimes methodically examine a patient and leave her undressed, cold, and embarrassed . We don't even bother to shut the curtain most of the time.

Since I had some medical experience, I often tried to explain the various procedures to patients and found myself frequently apologizing for the sometimes insensitive treatment. The patients really appreciated this as I received numerous letters of gratitude. Soon after starting as a volunteer I was offered a paid position in Patient Relations.

As a paid employee I found myself walking a fine line. I knew that I wanted to become a physician assistant, yet my job was mainly as a patient advocate. As a result, I often had to confront those, who may well have become my future colleagues, with patient complaints that were sometimes aimed at them. What I found was if I called patients by their names, instead of by body part, and if I quickly closed a curtain after an exam, that most of the staff started doing the same thing. This provided a much more comfortable environment for the patient and made my job a whole lot easier too.

SAMPLE B

Instead of joining the civilian arena after graduating from college, I decided to join the United States Air Force. I entered Officer's Training School not knowing what to expect, but with a lot of expectations. This service paid off in many ways. First, I learned to pay strict attention to detail. Second, the responsibility I had as a junior officer gave me the confidence to perform and accomplish many tasks working under less than ideal situations. Third, I learned the importance of teamwork and how to delegate responsibility in order to get the job done. Finally, I learned to always give one hundred percent since many people rely on me and trust my judgment. I left the Air Force with many accomplishments, including the Junior Officer of the Year award.

If you are a volunteer or working as a technician in the health care field, be careful not to profess that you know what it is like to be a physician assistant. On the other hand, try to let the reader know that you have thoroughly investigated the field and that you can write an intelligent and interesting essay.

IRREGULARITIES IN YOUR ACADEMIC RECORD

Most programs require you to send a copy of your college and high school transcripts along with your application. Many people will have excellent academic backgrounds. Many people will also have good academic backgrounds. Some applicants, however, will have a transcript which contains a few D's, F's, or W's. These people must address these grades somewhere on the application form. Some choose to use the essay itself; others will use the "additional comments" section. Choose whichever you prefer, but if you don't address this issue you may never get to the interview phase.

If you have many irregularities on your transcript, please consider re-taking the classes in which you did poorly. When you write about these ir-regularities, **do not make excuses.** Offer an explanation as best you can without sounding as if you are a "victim" of circumstance. Point out that you are aware of the deficiencies in your record and tell the reader what you have done about it. What have you learned as a result of your mistakes?

This gentleman explains why he was suspended from school in his freshman year.

> I was accepted to Weaver College on a baseball scholarship. At that time I was used to being a "star athlete" and having everything done for me. In my freshman year I paid more attention to playing baseball, and trying to fit in with the team, than I did to my studies. As a result, my grades suffered and I was suspended for the rest of the semester. That gave me a lot of time to think about which direction I was headed in. Yes, I came to college to play baseball, but my main goal was to get a good education so that I could some-day fulfill my dream of working in health care. Upon returning to school that next semester I promised myself that I would change my ways and give my education top priority. I worked extremely hard and have maintained a solid 3.3 grade point average since then. I also learned that it does not have to be all or nothing, as I continued playing baseball and volunteering at the local hospital.

The following is an example of a poor explanation for below average grades. The writer assumes no responsibility for her part in the deficiencies and this paragraph will reflect negatively on her as a mature, responsible candidate. She is what I call an "excusiologist."

> I would like to use this section of my application to write about some of the low grades I have received. I strongly feel that my transcripts do not provide an adequate representation of my ability to perform well as a physician assis-tant student. For example, in my sophomore year, I took organic chemistry with the same instructor for two semesters and received D's both times. The professor and I did not hit it off very well, and I feel that he held this against me when scoring tests and lab assignments. With regards to the "F" in psy-chology, my entire grade was based on a paper that we had to hand in at the end of the course. My paper was two days late because of my being away tak-ing care of my mother who was suffering from a serious heart illness. I notified the instructor before I left that my paper might be late. I assumed that it would be all right, but when I received my grade it was too late to do anything about it. I spoke with my guidance counselor, but he informed me that the syllabus clearly states that the final paper must be handed in on time to re-ceive a passing grade; there was nothing he could do. My attempts to contact my instructor and talk it over with her were also futile and the grade stands.
>
> As far as the rest of the low grades are concerned, I feel as though two main factors contributed to my deficiencies. First of all, I went to a very poor

YOU MUST EXPLAIN IRREGULARITIES IN YOUR ACADEMIC RECORD. DON'T BE AN EXCUSIOLOGIST!

high school. Many of the students were more interested in partying than studying. As a result, the teachers were frustrated and did not do a very good job trying to motivate the class. Once I got to college I had a lot of catching up to do and my grades suffered. In addition, I overloaded myself with science courses and labs in my junior year because I switched majors. I always had two or three lab reports to do per week, and this took up a great deal of my time that I would ordinarily spend studying. In my senior year, however, I really settled down and achieved a 3.5 average for the year.

This explanation is too lengthy and full of excuses. Readers of this essay are likely to put it to one side and go on to a more interesting candidate.

NON-TRADITIONAL BACKGROUND

MOST PA SCHOOL APPLICANTS ARE "NON-TRADITIONAL" AND MOST HAVE "TRANSFERABLE SKILLS."

Applicants may be non-traditional by virtue of age, race, medical experience, academic background, grade point average (GPA), or life experience. Too many applicants feel that they are at a disadvantage because of this. In reality, however, a student from a non-traditional background is sometimes a more interesting candidate than the traditional applicant. It all depends on how you present yourself, and your story, to the reader. You must learn to turn your own particular situation into a positive experience.

The following excerpt is from a young woman's essay who explains how her degree in dance and her work in massage therapy qualify her as a strong candidate.

> Through my degree in dance/kinesiology I learned of the many intricate movements the human body is capable of performing, as well as the limitations of our muscles, bones, and joints. Soon after graduating I opened a small practice as a massage therapist. I worked with a variety of patients and found that my best skill was listening intently to complaints and spending enough time with the patient to work them out. I continued to study anatomy and physiology in order to best serve my patients. I now have a longing to do more. I would like to build on what I have learned and begin to diagnose and treat patients in the medical arena. I am confident that my prior experience will aid me in this quest.

The above writer also does a great job demonstrating that she possesses "transferable skills." Although she has not worked directly in a clinical setting, she does a good job of telling the reader that the skills she has learned as a massage therapist will suit her well as a physician assistant.

LONG-TERM GOALS

You may be asked to comment on your future plans in your essay, or in the interview. It may be unrealistic for an applicant to know exactly what she wants to do when finishing school. If you do have some definite plans, however, and you have something substantial to say, then by all means mention it. But if you really have no definitive plans, which is fine, by the way, then tell the committee that you are exploring several options and wish to keep an open mind at this time. Once you finish your clinical training, you may have a better idea.

PERSONAL PHILOSOPHY

This can be a very dangerous area, and while we all have our own convictions about certain topics, it is always best to keep on the conservative side. If you can speak intelligently and maturely about a topic which may give the reader some more insight into you as a person, then it may be permissible to speak on the subject. Avoid controversy at all costs, however. The last thing that you want to do is get involved in a controversy.

RE-APPLICANTS

You should definitely write a completely new essay this year. Be sure to mention how you have grown and what you have learned since last year. Also, send in fresh letters of reference along with your application. You must show that you have made some positive changes since your last application.

When you sit down to write your second essay, other issues and concerns may arise. We recommend that you think about the following:

1. Your initial thoughts after receiving your letter of rejection.
2. How you felt and reacted after the disappointment wore off.
3. Did you call the director of the program (post-interview) and ask why you were not accepted?
4. Your reaction to the director's comments and your subsequent behavior.
5. What have you done since speaking with the program director?
6. Have you made any progress since your last application?
7. Have you had any significant changes in grades or work experiences?
8. Why are you now a better candidate than last year?

Now it is time to re-write your essay from a re-applicant's point of view. Focus on the last question, *Why are you now a better candidate than last year?*

EVOLUTION OF AN ESSAY

The following essay is a first draft from a young woman applying to PA school. After presenting the draft below, we will dissect it by paragraph and rewrite it so it is more effective.

When I was young; I vividly remember dressing up as a doctor for Halloween and dreaming of becoming one "when I grew up." At that early age, I viewed those in the health professions through rose colored glasses, as though I thought they would heroically heal people though an injection or a prescription. However, during a hospital internship my senior year, in high school, I realized that the OR is not always that miraculous center of recovery I had once envisioned. While observing a craniotomy, I watched a patient die on the operating table. I was shocked at the distance the health care team had, then realized that death was something inevitable that health care providers face everyday. The physicians, along with the rest of the health care team fulfilled their obligation; to try to cure the patient of a malignant brain tumor. It was then I learned that although modern medicine can prolong life, in the long run, it is death that wins because of the limitations of the human body. However, I decided that merely observing death impassively was beyond me, that I would wish to interact with the patients more intimately than the physician can.

After graduating high school, for two consecutive summers I interned for an orthopedic surgeon. Although I had seen PA's previously, the first time I really took note of one was outside the OR watching her comfort a patient just about to enter the OR. She was explaining exactly what was going to happen once the patient would enter the OR. I could tell that the patient deeply appreciated this extra attention he wouldn't have otherwise received. later, while reviewing the patient's chart prior to his surgery, I struck up a conversation with an orthopedic PA. As we chatted outside the OR, she asked me whether I planned to go to medical school. Though I had always known I wanted to work in the health care field, I was not sure that I really wanted to become a physician. The aspect of diagnosing and treating patients was what I wanted to do. However, I did not want to spend the next ten to twelve years of my life in school, nor did I seek the confinement and lack of family time a doctor experiences. As my new friend described her profession, I could discern her enthusiasm for it and her caring personality, both of which struck a responsive chord within me. Until I met this PA, I was unaware of how my character and the traits requisite for being a PA coincide.

Every chance I received, I took advantage of my opportunities to investigate the functions of a PA. More and more I became interested in the PA's ability not only to make decisions autonomously but to work as a team with other physicians and nurses. I relish the notion of interacting directly with my patients and help select the optimal way to comfort and cure them. I was also struck by the PA program's versatility and flexibility, which allow me to change specialties if I desire. Being an independent thinker, as well as a people oriented individual, I have concluded that I am well suited not just for the medical field but for a lifetime career as a PA.

I look forward to this fall to furthering my experience with PA's, when I will be shadowing a PA in the ER of Austin's Brackenridge Hospital. I know that further acquaintance with this position will enhance my understanding of what, I hope, my life's career and help prepare me for its rigors and rewards. Nevertheless, I am already positive that I have found my true calling in life and eagerly anticipate working together with my PA colleagues assisting others to return to the sometimes rock-strewn road to good health. because the operating room has always been my passion, I most likely will want to concentrate in that area, but as a highly receptive and open-minded person, I will be more than willing to change and focus in different spheres of health care if the occasion to do so arises.

In essence, my background in the medical field and witnessing many different procedures have convinced me that my lifetime dream can best come to reality through dedicating myself to a career as a PA.

L.L.

Paragraph #1. This young writer uses word pictures to try and make her essay more interesting. The problem is that her sentences are sometimes awkward and confuse the reader. She also, unintentionally, makes it sound as though the health care team is cold and uncaring instead of professional and objective. In addition, she uses abbreviations without first using the complete term. Finally, she speaks of death as being in competition with life; death is a part of life.

Paragraph #2. The opening sentence is awkward. She uses "PA's" instead of PAs. She assumes that the patient would not have received the proper attention were it not for the PA. She uses the colloquial expression, "chatted." She writes, ". . . nor did I seek the confinement and lack of family time a doctor experiences." In fact, one does not usually "seek" a negative. She also uses the improper tense at the beginning of this same sentence, ". . . I did not want to . . ." should be ". . . I do not want to . . ."

Paragraph #3. In the first sentence the writer needs to explain when and where she took advantage of her opportunities to investigate the functions of PAs. She also has a big problem with tense. Since she is describing how she wants to become a PA, she should be writing either in the conditional tense, or in the future tense, stating, "I was also struck by the PA program's versatility and flexibility, which **will** allow me to change specialties if I desire."

Paragraph #4. This paragraph has numerous spelling and grammatical errors. She also uses the colloquial term, "rock-strewn." She also becomes a little too subjective saying, ". . . as a highly receptive and open-minded person . . ."

Paragraph #5. Needs to be grammatically stronger without the participle "witnessing."

Here is the final version of the same essay.

> When I was a child, I vividly remember dressing up as a doctor for Halloween. At that early age I viewed those in the health profession through rose-colored glasses, as if I thought they would heroically heal people through an injection or with a prescription. However, during a hospital internship in my senior year in high school I realized that the operating room (OR) is not always the miraculous center of recovery I had envisaged. While observing a craniotomy I watched a patient die on the operating table. I was shocked that the health care team seemed to handle this with considerable objectivity and emotional distance, until I realized that death was an inevitability that health care providers face everyday. The physicians and other members of the health care team had fulfilled their obligation: to try to cure the patient of a malignant brain tumor. I learned that although modern medicine can prolong life, in the long run death is unavoidable because of the limitations of the human body. However, I decided that merely observing death impassively was beyond me and that I wanted to interact with patients more closely than a physician has the time to do.
>
> After graduating from high school, I interned for an orthopedic surgeon for two consecutive summers. Although I had seen PAs previously, the first time I really took note of one was outside the OR watching her comfort a patient just about to undergo a surgical procedure. The PA explained exactly what was going to happen to him once he entered the room. I could tell that the patient deeply appreciated this extra attention as he began to smile and his face became more relaxed.
>
> Later, while reviewing another patient's chart prior to her surgery, I began speaking with an orthopedic PA, Sherry. As we talked outside the holding area, she asked me whether I planned to go to medical school. Although I always knew I wanted to work in health care, I was not really sure that I wanted to become a physician. On the one hand I wanted the challenge of diagnosing and treating patients, but on the other hand I did not want to invest ten years of my life pursuing this goal. I also have plans of raising a family someday, and relish the idea of spending as much time as possible with them. As my new acquaintance described her profession, I could discern her enthusiasm for it and her caring personality, both of which struck a responsive chord in me. Until I met Sherry, I was unaware of how my character and the traits required for being a PA coincide.
>
> Every chance I received after that meeting, I took advantage of my opportunities to investigate the functions of PAs working in various fields. More and more, I became interested in the PA's ability not only to make decisions autonomously, but to work collaboratively with other members of the health care team. I look forward to being able to interact directly with my own patients and to, one day, be able to comfort them, and hopefully play a significant role in curing them, too. Being an independent thinker and working in a very versatile and flexible career are all very appealing to me.

This fall, I look forward to furthering my experience with PAs, when I will shadow a PA in the emergency room of Austin's Brackenridge Hospital. I am confident that further acquaintance with this position will enhance my understanding of what I hope will be my life's career and help prepare me for its rigors and rewards. Nevertheless, I am already positive that I have found my true calling in life, and eagerly anticipate working together with my PA colleagues assisting others to return on the sometimes difficult road to good health. Because the operating room is my passion, I will more than likely want to concentrate in surgery, but as a receptive and open-minded person, I will be willing to change and focus in different arenas of health care if the occasion to do so arises.

In essence, my background in the medical field and the fact that I have witnessed PAs working in various environments have convinced me that my lifetime dream can best come to fruition through dedicating myself to a career as a PA.

My other recommendation to this candidate was to provide examples of other skills, collaborative work experiences, and organizational duties or functions.

ESSAYS THAT WORKED

(SAMPLE #1)

"Attach to this application a typewritten narrative of not more than two pages, explaining where you learned of the PA profession, what factors or influences led you to this career choice, and how you expect to fulfill your goals as a physician associate."

For four years in the middle 1970s I was a Navy Corpsman, providing direct medical care to more than 400 marines, often in conditions of urgency and with little or no supervision. During this time I was exposed to the drama and trauma associated with medical care on a day-to-day basis. I learned how to work under conditions of limited or imperfect information and how to maintain composure under stress. Most importantly, I felt firsthand the profound satisfaction that comes from successfully delivering medical care.

After an Honorable Discharge from the Navy in 1979, I worked in the Yale–New Haven Hospital as an emergency room technician. During this time I had a chance to develop my skills as a team worker in a collaborative environment. This experience significantly broadened my view of disease and death, as the majority of our patients were not healthy young males as they tended to be in the military. I saw the direct effects of disease on infants, children, adolescents, adults, and elderly people of all ages, ethnic backgrounds, and socioeconomic conditions.

At Yale–New Haven, I worked closely with a physician associate. This was the first time I had ever been exposed to this career. His obvious technical expertise and medical knowledge were impressive. However, the profession was far less developed than it is today. I left the emergency room knowing that I wanted to pursue my career interests in health care, but unsure of which route to follow. I then decided to earn a four-year degree in Chemistry.

During my junior year in college, my career plans were changed drastically by the birth of my first child. Since I did not wish to continue to head a household as the proverbial "starving student," I decided upon graduating to rejoin the military, in this case the Air Force. This represented a degree of security to me for the time being.

For the past several years I have been an industrial salesperson. It has been quite rewarding from the point of view of allowing me to provide a good standard of living for myself and my family. However, it does not give the deep satisfaction I receive from my hospital volunteer work. I have the feeling that the products I sell could be sold by anyone, but that service as a health professional is a genuine honor and calling.

So, what, at my age and professional level, is the best way to become a health professional? To attempt to go to medical school would be an enormous investment of time and money. I have considered nursing or acting as a nurse practitioner, but I am more interested in the technical and diagnostic aspects of medicine and the close partnership with a physician that being a physician associate can give.

In my deliberations over making this career choice, I have talked extensively with physicians, physician associates, and other health care professionals. I have taken further coursework and done well. One of the reasons that the profession of physician associate appeals to me as a long-term career choice is the opportunity to directly influence people in a positive way. Specifically, I am referring to the importance of continuing to emphasize in a strong but helpful way the basics of preventive medicine. In the past year a relative and two close friends died from preventable diseases. This has dramatically shown me the responsibility a caregiver has in encouraging habits which prolong and improve the quality of life.

I have come to see and believe strongly in the concept that good medicine does not only come from bottles and boxes, but also from the heart and feelings of the caregiver. To be truly effective as a physician associate, I will have to excel in technical ability and medical knowledge, but also as a communicator. Very few people can, in the course of their work, help save or significantly prolong a life. As a physician associate, I will have the opportunity of taking a minute to talk about why stop smoking or go on a diet. This to me is a true measure of career satisfaction.

One of the most valuable aspects of my experience has been the opportunity to work with and for outstanding individuals. These people are not only scientifically rigorous with information, but extremely humane in their dealings with others, both colleagues and patients. One such individual is a physician associate with whom I work at St. Raphael's Hospital. She is energetic, positive, personable, seems to always have a moment and a good word for everybody. Above all, she is a total professional and earns by her daily efforts the respect of those she works with.

The Physician Associate Program is an ideal way to realize career ambitions in health care. Physician associates have the chance to act at a significant level of intervention with patients without needing to invest the years and years of training that becoming a physician would require.

If given the opportunity, I plan to use my physician associate training to return to the Emergency Room in a newly enhanced role. This, to me, is where so much of the opportunity exists to practice the skills I have and will develop. I enjoy the direct contact with people, the fast-changing environment, and most of all the chance to directly work with and help people who are in serious need. With the AIDS epidemic, the prevalence of teen violence, and the enormous substance abuse problems today, I am sure that there will be more need than ever for skilled, competent individuals to assist in this critical area.

A.J.R.

(SAMPLE #2)

"Tell the committee what factors led you to choose a career as a physician assistant, and how you have prepared yourself for this role."

My decision to seek a career in medicine was influenced by several personal and work-based experiences. However, it was my grandfather, a very important person in my life, who played a significant role in finalizing my career choice. Shortly after my thirteenth birthday, he was hospitalized with a heart attack. He subsequently underwent heart surgery and suffered a stroke in the immediate post-operative period. I felt overwhelmed by the fact that no one seemed to be able to do anything to help him. One day while I sat at his bedside I realized that I wanted to get involved in medicine, and I promised him that I would work hard to be able to help others get well. The next week he died, and I became more determined than ever to make a difference by caring for others.

Over the last several years, my interest in becoming a physician assistant has been strengthened by my extracurricular and work activities. While in high school I worked as a unit clerk, part-time, on a busy surgical floor. It was here that I was briefly introduced to the work of PAs. My duties consisted of answering the phone, ordering lab tests, and, at times, interacting with the patients. As a result of this exposure, I became familiar with medical terminology, learned about the health care "team" concept, and played a significant role in recruiting volunteers to our floor to spend time with our patients. During the summer of 1990, I received my first "hands-on" experience and my first direct working contact with PAs. I worked as a technician in the emergency room alongside nurses, doctors, technicians, and PAs. I collected and measured vital signs, obtained short medical histories, assisted in trauma cases, and sometimes just held a patient's hand to comfort her. It was here that I learned that the practice of medicine is as much about good care-giving as it is about the appropriate drug therapy.

In 1992, while studying chemistry at Southern University, I participated in numerous extracurricular activities, thus enhancing my leadership and interpersonal skills. These activities provided situations in which I was allowed to exercise my capabilities as president, vice-president, treasurer, and secretary. For instance, in my role as president of the Spanish Club, I initiated activities such as a winter coat drive for inner city Hispanic children, and worked with a team of community leaders and students to achieve our goal of collecting over 1000 coats.

I have also been involved in other activities which have given me the opportunity to help those who are socio-economically disadvantaged and unable to care for themselves. This volunteer work ranged from working at the Saint Ann's soup kitchen and reading to the blind, to holding and feeding "crack" babies in the Newborn Intensive Care Unit at Michener Hospital. As a result of these experiences, I learned to reach out to others and help make a positive change in their lives. I also made quite a few new friends along the way. At Michener Hospital, I also worked on the crisis hot-line where my responsibilities were to be an attentive, confident listener and to provide the caller with reference information pertinent to the inquiry. Through this experience I have gained confidence in dealing with crisis situations.

During my senior year at Southern, I was employed by the local Veteran's Hospital as a cardiac rehabilitation aide. I worked very closely with patients either recovering from bypass surgery or from heart attacks. I walked with patients, counseled them on proper nutrition, and helped develop an exercise regimen for the "Take Heart" program. This experience improved my ability to listen to patients and to teach them at the same time.

Presently, I am a volunteer with the Orange County Fire Department. I work as an EMT. This experience is teaching me how to work under extreme conditions of stress.

My desire to become a physician assistant is sincere and founded on a working knowledge of the role of PAs. I am committed to doing whatever is necessary to achieve my goal.

D.K.

(SAMPLE # 3)

This applicant was accepted to every program that she applied to: Duke, Yale, Northeastern, and George Washington. She has a rich cultural and ethnic history, and she uses her experiences very effectively.

The majority of my extracurricular activities fall under the following categories:

A) Music

I began to take flute lessons in 1974 at the age of seven and at thirteen also began violin lessons. I have become quite accomplished on both instruments and have played in various musical ensembles. Presently I play first-flute in the Stratford, Connecticut Community Band, of which I am the youngest member, and first-flute in the Fairfield University Flute Choir, which I helped organize in 1986. From 1981 to 1983, I played first violin in the Bridgeport, Connecticut Youth Symphony, the Norwalk, Connecticut Youth Symphony, and the Sherwood Orchestra. Other ensembles include the Fairfield University Chamber Orchestra and groups annually assembled by my music teachers to regularly perform for residents of convalescent homes. Over the years I have also played in local bands and done solo performances at various private parties and organizational functions.

B) Ethnic Activities

My home life is quite unique in that my parents are immigrants from Czecho-Slovakia and as a result I am able to speak, read, and write the Slovak language fluently. I greatly value my Slovak heritage and culture, and thus a great deal of my time is spent on ethnic activities.

From 1986 to 1987, I served as the General Chairman of the centennial celebration of the St. John Nepomucene Society, the oldest Slovak fraternal society in New England. My leadership abilities were strengthened by this event for, having been given a free hand by the society officers, I directed all arrangements and preparations. This year-long activity culminated in a successful weekend program highlighted by religious services and a banquet attended by over 360 people.

In August 1988, I was selected to be a delegate to the 32nd National Convention of the "First Slovak Wreath of the Free Eagle," a national Slovak–American fraternal society which was organized in 1986. At the convention I was appointed to serve on the by-laws committee and as assistant secretary of the convention. I was also honored by being elected to the office of Supreme Youth Director. Not only was I the youngest member in attendance at the convention, but also the youngest, in the ninety-two year history of the organization, to be elected to the Board of Directors.

To conserve and perpetuate our Slovak culture and traditions, the Slovak societies also sponsor weekly radio programs which I help produce. At WWPT, Westport, Connecticut, I help produce and coordinate the "Slovak Alliance Program," which presents traditional folk songs from Slovakia. At WSHU, Fairfield, Connecticut, I help produce and coordinate "Music from Slovakia," which presents both classical and traditional music written or performed by Slovak composers and ensembles.

C) Work Experience

To help finance my education I work throughout the year. From September 1984 to May 1987, I was a counter worker at a dry-cleaning establishment, averaging thirty-five hours per week during the school year and fifty hours per week during the summer months. A most enjoyable aspect of this job was the constant contact I had with the public. The interaction with various people certainly sharpened my social skills.

From June 1987 to present, I have worked for a dermatologist and average twenty-five hours per week. As a medical assistant at the physician's office, I have gotten hands-on experience and insight into how a physician works in a private practice and how a medical office is run. My duties range from reception to assisting the doctor or nurse.

As a receptionist, I log in patients and make them feel comfortable and answer questions regarding medications, services, and surgeries. The clerical aspect includes typing referral letters and reports, billing, and handling health insurance claims. I often assist the doctor with minor surgery, which also includes preparing specimens for the Pathology lab and charting. Most interesting has been my observation of and assistance with hair transplantation surgery, microscopic work, and phlebotomy necessary for the "Fibrel" injections used in scar and wrinkle treatment. At the office I also make up solutions of Minoxidil used in the treatment of hair loss, monitor the blood pressure of Minoxidil patients, and make up a moisturizing cream with Tretinoin (Retin A) used to prevent skin wrinkles and acne.

In addition, I am presently a teaching assistant for the Freshman Biology lab at Fairfield University, a volunteer therapist's assistant for a program for handicapped children, and will soon be certified to perform cardiopulmonary resuscitation (CPR). My experiences in the health care field are quite varied and have not only expanded my medical knowledge but have also provided me with valuable practical experience.

D) Miscellaneous

My other community activities include working as a volunteer at the Easter Seals Rehabilitation Center, Bridgeport, Connecticut, where I work with young children suffering mental and physical handicaps. I also volunteer my time at the Merton House soup kitchen, Bridgeport, Connecticut, which provides food and clothing for the poor and homeless.

E) Why I Want to Pursue a Career in Medicine

Sometimes a person experiences one significant event which changes her life and outlook. For me it occurred in 1978 when my father suffered a severe skull fracture due to a fall from a ladder. He remained in a coma for five days but, luckily, he completely recovered from his injuries. This close encounter with death left me with a greater appreciation of, and respect for, life. Most importantly, however, this experience gave me an incentive. I am forever indebted to God and to the physicians for caring for my father's life, and my career choice is my way of repaying this debt. I am willing to make many more sacrifices in order to achieve my goal, and if I can help others just as my father was helped, and if I can inspire someone just as I was inspired, I know all of my work and sacrifice will not be in vain. This calling comes from deep within me, and I am confident that I can and will achieve my goal.

L.H.

(SAMPLE #4)

The focus of this candidate's essay is on making a career change. She is also an "older" applicant.

My first exposure to the Physician Associate profession was in 1982 when I was treated for a minor medical problem by a PA at CHCP. I asked the universal question of "What is a PA?" and spoke with the PA briefly about his work. Since then I have had regular contact with PAs through my health insurance providers. Once I seriously considered the PA profession for myself, I read professional journals, the Physician Assistant Journal and the Journal of the American Academy of Physician Assistants, and talked with PAs to learn more about the profession.

I am currently looking to make a change in my career. The last couple of years have been a time for reflection and change, with a focus on reviewing my career objectives. I have come to the conclusion that I want to be involved in a career that:

- ▶ has a bright future
- ▶ is directly involved with people
- ▶ is in the medical arena
- ▶ meets my need for continuing education and opportunity for change
- ▶ will utilize my past life/work experiences and skills

The Physician Associate profession meets all of these criteria.

There is no question as to the viability of the profession. Certainly, the creation of a national health care system which demands affordable health care will only increase that need. Indicators predict that the PA profession will be growing for the next decade and beyond. I still have another 20–25 years of work ahead of me and want my next profession to be one that will offer a lot of opportunity.

My need to be involved with people has been lifelong. I have been able to meet this need through volunteer experiences as well as through the evolution of my career. In my first position as Horticulture Manager, I worked directly with individuals who have differing needs, planning and providing vocational rehabilitation programs. I met with their families and, at times, found myself in situations which were emotional and challenging. As Personnel Director, I have worked with staff, applicants, and volunteers in areas of hiring, firing, terminal illness, addictions, work-related injuries, and performance issues.

Within this area I have had to make tough decisions without letting my personal bias interfere. With these previous experiences, I have developed strong interpersonal skills which will be a substantial asset to me as a PA.

I now find that I want to become involved with people at a more critical level, focusing on their good health and wellness. My original career interests took me in many different directions. I was very interested in physical therapy and the human sciences but also had a strong attraction to horticulture and the plant sciences. My decision to enter the field of horticulture therapy came when I learned that I could combine my two areas of interest. After 5 years of providing hands-on services in a vocational rehabilitation environment, I felt the need to become part of the administrative team and entered graduate school to study organization and management. Now that I have been in administration for 8 years, I find that my interests are pulling me into the medical field again.

As my life progresses, I have observed in myself the need for a profession that offers a diverse array of opportunities. In addition to the diversity of a PA's career options, I find it revitalizing to be in a profession that requires continuing education. The prospect of a career with broad possibilities and education expansion is both attractive and motivational.

Changing my career will only make sense if I can utilize my past work experiences and skills. It is in this area that I feel I will be able to give the most back to the PA profession. In my 15 years with SARAH, I have developed and implemented both the horticulture and personnel departments from infancy. I now am in the process of implementing yet another new department for SARAH, quality evaluation, for which I will be the Director. As the PA profession continues to flourish, there will be a need for people with an administrative and management background such as mine to create and administer the growing number of programs and services PAs will be providing.

I consider returning to school as an "older student" a very exciting opportunity. The time I spent at Antioch New England Graduate School was one of the most stimulating periods of my life, thus far. The experience of working 40 hours per week at SARAH and going to school nights in Hartford and weekends in Keene, New Hampshire, lifted me to a level of energy and motivation that was both stimulating and rewarding. I believe that I will be very successful entering _____ PA program, with its intensive and rigorous curriculum, given my success at Antioch. I look forward to the challenge with excitement and confidence.

At this point in my life, a career move requires much thought and consideration. After reassessing my career options, I feel that this is the time to make a move. The Physician Associate profession will bring me back to my original interest in medicine and meet all of my career objectives. By combining my successful educational and work history with my original desire and aptitude in the physical sciences, I am confident that you will find me to be an excellent candidate for your program.

I look forward to having the opportunity to meet with you in an interview for student selection to further discuss my interest in _____ Physician Associate program.

T.S.

What follows are several annotated essay examples, and a selection of paragraphs from essays. These examples may further help you when constructing your own narrative.

ANNOTATED ESSAY 1

Charles Boelter

The first time I can recall meeting a Physician Assistant was in the emergency room of Martin Army Community Hospital, on Fort Benning, Georgia. I was a private, going through basic infantry training and happened to be clumsy enough to fall from the top of the forty-foot rope climb on the obstacle course. I knew he was an officer, but he obviously was neither a doctor nor a nurse. He pulled a large piece of wood from under my thumbnail, and sent me for some x-rays. He determined that I was not mortally wounded, and released me to my unit.

I managed to survive basic training, and eventually I wound up as a paratrooper in the Eighty-Second Airborne Division. Throughout the course of my enlistment, I was able to spend a considerable amount of time with our battalion PA. I learned what he did and what options his profession provided him. When the time came for me to leave active duty, I was beginning to think about the Physician Assistant profession as a career path.

I have wanted a career in medicine for as long as I can remember. I am sure this is because of my father, and the stories I have heard about him. He learned the intricacies of medicine in school, but he was born with the innate ability to care for, and about, people.

We lived in a small town, amidst a million acres of corn, in rural Illinois. My father practiced from a small office that was actually our converted garage. From this office he took care of the people in our town on the surrounding farms, and those in the nearby communities. Less than one month after my brother was born, our father left on a house call from which he never returned. He died that night, leaving his sons a legacy of caring and competency that I hear about to this day. My brother never felt the calling of the medical profession as strongly as I have, so he offered encouragement and support to help me achieve my goals. His encouragement stopped when he was killed shortly after I left the military. His death left me as the only one to follow in my father's footsteps.

OPENING PARAGRAPH USES A SCENARIO WITH IMMEDIACY TO GAIN THE ATTENTION OF THE READER.

OUTLINES INTEREST IN THE PA PROFESSION.

IDENTIFIES A MORE DEEPLY FELT MOTIVATION.

STRONG PERSONAL AND EMOTIONAL EXPERIENCES ARE STATED WITH RESTRAINT.

My life has prepared me for a career as a Physician Assistant in many ways. I believe that, like my father, I have an innate ability to care about people and what happens to them. I want to help make positive changes in their lives much as my father did. Being a soldier matured me and taught me self-confidence. Being a leader taught me to be responsible for myself, and for my subordinates. I learned not only how to make decisions, but also to recognize the consequences those decisions might have. My work as a medical assistant has given me a better understanding of how the medical team works together to satisfy patient needs. It has exposed me to clinical decision making and the complexities of modern medicine. I have seen first hand the role Physician Assistants fulfill in the medical community, and how they fit into the team approach to care, by shadowing them in various settings. I believe I have been given the character and the ability to become a competent Physician Assistant.

My strongest desire in life is to experience the joys and rigors of a profession in medicine much as my father did. I have the ability and desire to help people, but I need the tools to do this. Becoming a Physician Assistant will give me the tools I need to take the next step in my career. This is the path I am on, and it is where I can offer the most for those who need help.

ANNOTATED ESSAY 2

Yvonne Gonzalez

My interest in becoming a Physician Associate (PA) is rooted in the desire to provide quality health care to the underprivileged—whose health care needs I have perceived to be acute in the course of my volunteer work. As Social Justice Coordinator for my parish, I organized volunteer efforts at a number of facilities: pediatric clinics and orphanages in Baja, California, the L.A. Mission and the Catholic Worker (a soup kitchen and free clinic in L.A.). I also represented the parish in a 10-day, 250-mile walk-athon from Santa Barbara to Tijuana to raise money for a child welfare agency. I have never felt so much satisfaction in my career achievements as compared to the gratification I derive from working with the underprivileged. Their acute health care needs prompted my desire to become involved in a professional capacity. I felt frustrated, however, because I did not want to become a physician and just could not see myself in any of the allied health careers. It was not until I learned of the Physician Associate profession that I realized I could fulfill my dream of working in public health at a significant level of medical intervention without having to train for 8 or more years.

I first learned of Physician Associates when my father had a double by-pass in 1994 and his post-operative care was managed by his cardiologist's staff PA, Helen. When she explained her role to me, I was impressed with the scope of her responsibilities and sensed that this might be the opportunity I had been seeking. Not long after I met Helen, I began shadowing Ted Braunstein, a PA in the Emergency Department of Mount Sinai Medical Center. I was impressed by his clinical knowledge, compassion, and aptitude for patient education. I was also surprised to see the degree of autonomy given Ted by the attending physicians. We worked out a pact: Ted would answer all of my questions and I would help him obtain histories and physicals on Spanish-speaking patients. I soon found myself assisting the patient representatives when they were short-handed. It wasn't long before I was gloving up to help steady patients as Ted performed suturing or lumbar punctures. Next, the technicians taught me how to draw blood, insert Foley catheters, and take vital measurements. Even after over 1500 hours, I am still amazed at the fascinating array of patients and clinical challenges every shift offers.

EVIDENCE OF SELF-REFLECTION AND UNDERSTANDING OF HIS OWN SKILLS AND ABILITIES.

RE-CAPS HIS REASONS FOR WANTING TO BECOME A PA IN A SUCCINCT CONCLUSION.

CLEAR OPENING SENTENCE WHICH PAVES THE WAY FOR FURTHER SUPPORTING EVIDENCE.

STRONG HISTORY OF VOLUNTEER WORK AND UNDERSTANDING OF SOCIAL JUSTICE ISSUES.

FOCUSES THE READER ON HER INITIAL INTEREST IN THE PROFESSION AND THEN BUILDS ON HOW IT DEVELOPED FURTHER INTO A LIFELONG GOAL.

USE OF HER OWN BACKGROUND AND LANGUAGE SKILLS TO IMPROVE PATIENT ACCESS TO CARE.

SPECIFICALLY LISTS THE SKILLS SHE ACQUIRED.

CLEAR VISION OF WHERE SHE
WANTS TO BE IN THE FUTURE.

USES A NEW SLANT ON HER
SKILLS TO CONSOLIDATE
THE ESSAY.

STRONG, UNUSUAL BEGINNING
PARAGRAPH LINKED TO THE
DESIRE TO STUDY MEDICINE.

EFFECT OF A PERSONAL
EXPERIENCE WHICH BECOMES A
TURNING POINT.

ANOTHER KEY TURNING POINT.

WORK OUTCOMES CLEARLY
STATED.

If given the opportunity, I plan to use my PA training to work in public health. Ideally, I would like to divide my time between an urban tertiary care facility and a rural clinic. Working in such diverse settings will, I feel, provide me with a strong clinical foundation and the opportunity for continuing education that will benefit both patient populations. Serving those in serious need will fulfill a lifelong goal and doing so in a PA capacity will allow me to utilize the analytical, communication, and time management skills I have acquired in my career thus far. My decision to become a PA is based on a working knowledge of the role of the PA, and I am committed to making the necessary sacrifices to achieve this goal.

ANNOTATED ESSAY 3

Norman deDios

I have always been fascinated by the mysteries of nature. While my boyhood friends admired Batman, I idolized Jacques Cousteau. To me, he represented man's unrelenting desire to explore the unknown, while demonstrating a deep respect for the natural order of living things. As a child, I consumed countless books on science and spent hours watching documentaries trying to understand the hows and whys of life. I even went so far as to set up my own "pet shop" in our basement which eventually contained one hundred tropical fish, ranging from a feisty red-eyed South American manguenese to a two-foot-long silver arrowana. It is this innate curiosity that has evolved into and become the foundation of my desire to study medicine.

My interest in the natural world took a personal and painful turn when I was awakened to the reality of human suffering during my sophomore year at Providence College. At that time, my father suffered a major heart attack, for which he required quadruple bypass surgery and a four-week stay in hospital. It was frightening to see the man who always seemed invincible to me lying in a hospital attached to so many machines. My father's illness forced me to redefine my role in the family and I suddenly found myself at its head. During this time I traveled regularly from Providence to New Haven to look after my father and provide support to my mother and siblings. Unfortunately, this sudden shift of responsibility and unfamiliar stress was reflected in my poor grades. The fragility of life and the importance of family became clear to me, and I realized that this difficult period would serve as a transition point toward a new level of maturity, a maturity that strengthened my ability to persevere and heightened my feelings of compassion and concern for others.

My work experience in health care began with a summer job as a Laboratory Assistant in the Blood Chemistry Laboratory of The Hospital of St. Raphael. My responsibilities included keeping records of blood specimens as well as interacting directly with physicians and other members of the hospital staff. The following summer, I was employed as an Operating Room Aide in the Ambulatory Surgery Unit of Yale–New Haven Hospital, where contact with patients on a personal level was a new and rewarding experience. My job gave me the opportunity to interact with patients before their surgery and also upon their discharge. It was extremely gratifying to know that the support I offered these patients was not only reassuring but also greatly appreciated. I have always felt a tremendous amount of self-reward knowing that I made a difference in a person's life, simply by showing them I cared. It was this personal time with patients that proved to be the most satisfying aspect of my job at Yale–New Haven and further motivated me to pursue a career in the health sciences.

After graduating from college, I accepted a position as a research assistant at Yale University School of Medicine, Department of OB/GYN. Working closely with Drs. Aydin Arici and Ibrahim Sozen on their leiomyoma research, I aided in the completion of their study on the effects of growth factor-B1 on myometrial tumors. Our work will be published in the near future. After completing my work with Drs. Arici and Sozen, I was given the opportunity to work with David Keefe, also of Yale's OB/GYN Department. I thoroughly enjoyed my time with Dr. Keefe due to his confidence in me to work unsupervised and because of the relationship we formed as I occasionally accompanied him throughout his busy day seeing patients. It was with Dr. Keefe that I gained an understanding and appreciation for the intimacy and trust patients have in their health care provider.

After leaving Yale, I continued to work in the field of research as a Laboratory Assistant in the Department of Molecular Genetics at New York Medical College. This laboratory was involved in the identification of the gene that causes ataxia telangiectasia, a neuromuscular disease that strikes young children. My responsibilities included cataloging daily blood specimens and isolating DNA for gene identification. Although my role was a small one, it was gratifying to know that my work may aid others in eventually finding a cure for this disease.

While I enjoyed my research, I missed the personal contact I had with patients. This led me to spend this past summer shadowing physician assistants in the Cardiothoracic Unit at The Hospital of St. Raphael, which rekindled my interest in clinical medicine. This experience has clarified my image of a physician assistant's role in health care, as well as given me a better understanding of where I hope to be in this field. My interest in patient care has been further enhanced by my current volunteer work with Yale–New Haven Hospital Elder-Life Program. This position allows me to work one-on-one with geriatric patients and has given me hands-on experience in the health care field. I also feel that volunteer work continues to develop techniques for communicating and interacting with patients that I will use in my career as a physician assistant.

Another area in which I have been able to refine my interpersonal skills has been through my involvement in music. Ten years ago, my friends and I formed a band in which we all continue to perform. As the keyboard player, a vocalist, and a guitarist, I realize that the ability to share and relate ideas is essential to being a successful and unified group. Through music, I have learned the value of patience, cooperation, and understanding, and strive to utilize these qualities in everyday life.

I believe that the adversities I have faced have helped me to mature, and I regard them as growing stages in my life. These events have affected me because I genuinely do care about others, and they have shown me how committed and determined I am. I sincerely believe that I now possess the qualities to become a responsible, compassionate, and caring physician assistant. Therefore, I refuse to let these obstacles discourage me and to this day I am continuing my education as well as my involvement in health care. I look forward to using my newly found reservoir of strength toward a lifelong career in medicine. My experiences in health care, and my interactions with physician assistants have only strengthened my resolve. I know that as time passes, I can use my experiences, both positive and negative to become a truly competent physician assistant.

EXAMPLES OF ESSAY EXTRACTS

OPENING PARAGRAPHS

Imagine waking every day of the year at four o'clock in the morning to care for one hundred head of dairy cattle. This is what my wife Carla and I have done for the past seventeen years. . . .

Bradford Phillips

LEARNING FROM OTHERS.

REMINDS THE READER OF ONE OF THE KEY FACTORS FOR HIM IN WISHING TO BECOME A PA.

GOOD EXAMPLE OF TRANSFERABLE SKILLS — THOSE SKILLS ACQUIRED IN ANOTHER AREA WHICH WILL BE USEFUL IN THE PA PROFESSION.

CLEAR REITERATION OF WHAT HE HAS SAID BEFORE WITH A SLIGHTLY DIFFERENT FOCUS.

During the past years, I have worked with or shadowed four exceptional Physician Assistants who have given me valuable insight to the PA profession. As I worked with these health care providers, I analyzed their skills and qualities and inventoried their commonalities. Besides maintaining a high level of technical proficiency, each of them is a superior team leader, outstanding communicator, and creative problem solver. My formal education in psychology and my personal experiences have provided me with an opportunity to develop those three vital qualities.

Amy Fritsch

The inextricable relationship between health and mental health has intrigued me for over fourteen years. As a teenager, I watched programs on public television about the etiology of psychotic disorders. After graduating from high school, I decided to follow my natural interests into the world of health care, earning degrees in mental health, psychology, and social work. With each educational milestone I have gained knowledge and experience that has enhanced my understanding of how to help others in need.

Barbara Ann Slusher

EXAMPLES OF A LEARNING EXPERIENCE WHICH HAD AN IMPACT ON AN INDIVIDUAL IN SHAPING HIS/HER ASPIRATIONS

A few years ago I had occasion to reassess where I was in life, and where I had expected to be at this point. I found that the two did not match, and in fact bore little resemblance to each other. It was time to make up my own mind about where and how I spend the rest of my life. The task then became one of determining what track I wanted my life to be on, and how I was going to get there. One of the steps in my search, led me to volunteer on the Neurology/Neurosurgery Nursing Unit at the George Washington University Medical Center—the first volunteer they had ever had. I quickly realized I not only felt very comfortable in the medical environment, but had also found a piece of what was missing in my life. Volunteering was good, and quite rewarding, but not nearly enough. I needed to be working in a medical field full time, and be in a position to provide patient care.

Jean Caldwell

The most poignant experience of my career that truly sparked my interest in medicine was my experience as a counselor in a methadone maintenance program. Our treatment team noticed marked improvements in the physical and mental health of our clients after only a short period of methadone treatment. It seemed that heroin addiction was a disease easily treated with methadone. What was confusing, however, was the high rate of relapse for clients who had successfully detoxified from the methadone after years of stable treatment.

Why did clients with such a positive prognosis and years of treatment relapse? We found that many factors influenced a client's ability to remain abstinent from drugs: lifestyle, HIV status, family history, socioeconomic status, et cetera. The relation between these factors was very complex. We could not treat just the physical aspect of the addiction and hope to be successful. For me, this learning experience underlined the fact that disease is not one dimensional. The best treatment approach is one that encompasses the physical, mental, and socio-emotional aspects of the individual in their environment.

Barbara Ann Slusher

. . . Although I had various responsibilities at the clinic, what stands out most in my mind was the time I spent listening, counseling, and teaching patients, and the tremendous satisfaction that came from this interaction. One woman I remember came in to see the internist. After a thorough exam and some laboratory tests, the doctor told her that she had diabetes and was going to have to begin insulin therapy. I translated since she spoke only Spanish and could not understand what the doctor was saying. She only asked a few questions and seemed very hesitant and frightened about her future. We reassured her that she was in good hands and we would all be there to support her with the steps she needed to take. A few days later she returned to learn about diabetes management and insulin injections, and again I translated for her. For both the nurse and me it was challenging because she was apprehensive and doubtful that she was going to be able to manage everything by herself. We reassured her that although it was going to be difficult in the beginning, she could do it. We sat with her as she practiced the various tasks, from testing her blood sugar level and giving herself an injection to documenting everything in her journal. After about an hour she was ready to go home, feeling more comfortable with her daily routine. As she left, she took my hand and thanked me for my patience and support, telling me what a good person I was. It seemed strange that she would thank me for this, but her gratitude showed me how important it is to take the time to listen, counsel, and support patients.

Katherine Coleman

EXAMPLE OF A STRONG CONCLUSION

These volunteer experiences have crystallized the challenges, rewards, and frustrations of being a health care provider, as well as the shortcomings of health care in the United States. These diverse environments have augmented my studies in public health, and have provided me with concrete examples of how individuals can benefit from caring, sensitive providers, and how communities suffer when adequate health care services are not available or affordable. As a Physician Assistant I will be poised to deliver health care services to under-served urban populations, and I will demonstrate compassion and sensitivity. Furthermore, the intensive, rigorous, PA program at . . . will enable me to execute this career change effectively and efficiently.

Lynn R. Fryer

WORK HISTORY SHEET

Employer name: _____

Address: _____

Phone #: _____

Full time:_____   Part-time: _____

Dates of Employment: From:_____   To: _____

Job Title:_____

Job Description: (3 sentences or less)_____

_____

_____

_____

_____

Skills utilized: _____

Awards/citations: _____

Other information: _____

MEDICAL EXPERIENCE SHEET

Employer name: _____

Address:_____

Phone #: _____

months worked: Full time:_____   Part time: _____

Dates of employment: _____

Job title:(3 sentences or less) _____

_____

_____

_____

_____

Skills utilized (phlebotomy, vital signs, physical exams):_____

_____

Awards/citations:_____

Describe your most memorable patient (3 sentences or less):

_____

_____

_____

_____

Other information: _____

HIGH SCHOOL INFORMATION SHEET

High school attended: _____

Address:_____

Dates attended: From _____ to _____

Major course of study: _____

GPA: _____

Team sports: _____

Clubs: _____

Awards/honors: _____

Volunteer work: _____

Other: _____

COLLEGE INFORMATION SHEET

College/University attended:_____

Address:_____

Dates: _____

Major:_____

Highest degree obtained: _____

GPA: _____

Team sports: _____

Clubs: _____

Volunteer work: _____

Awards/honors: _____

Did you work?:   yes___   no___

List one person who you can contact for a good reference: _____

_____

Scholarships: _____

Other: _____

VOLUNTEER WORK

Volunteer description: _____

Why this position?: _____

Address:_____

Point of contact: _____

How long?:_____

Awards/letters of appreciation: _____

Most memorable patient/experience: _____

List one person who will write a good reference for you: _____

_____

MILITARY SERVICE

Branch of service: _____

Dates of service:_____

Discharge type: (honorable, general, etc.)_____

Where stationed?: _____

Job title (M.O.S.):_____

Supervisor: _____

Awards/ribbons/medals: _____

Special schools/training: _____

Did you attend college in the military?:_____

What did you learn from the experience? (teamwork, discipline, etc.): _____

_____

FOREIGN LANGUAGE

Do you speak a foreign language?:_____

What language: _____

How did you learn the language?: _____

TRAVEL

Where to?: _____

When?: _____

What did you learn from the experience?: _____

SPECIAL AWARDS/CITATIONS

Award type: _____

Why received?: _____

When received?: _____

Given by: _____

What did you do to get it?: _____

Finally, you rush to the mailbox, open the letter from the PA program you're applying to, and read, "Congratulations, out of 500 applicants this year, the committee would like to interview you . . ." After you let out a scream, you relax and realize that your chances of getting accepted have just risen drastically. After the exhilaration wears off, you will begin to get a little nervous and some doubt may creep in. Don't be alarmed, you have what it takes to get the interview; now it's time to shine.

This chapter will discuss how to improve your communication skills and use them to your advantage in an interview situation.

HIGH-IMPACT COMMUNICATION

WINNING THROUGH HIGH-IMPACT COMMUNICATION

Charisma: defined in Funk and Wagnalls' dictionary as **extraordinary personal power or charm.** To some it comes naturally, but more often than not it must be learned. Charisma is the result of a series of behaviors through which someone has a powerful and positive impact on others. In this chapter we will teach you how to develop your own personal charisma in order to build a bridge to credibility and trust.

General H. Norman Schwarzkopf, John Madden, Jane Pauley, Katie Couric, and Elizabeth Dole all have charisma. They move beyond facts, figures, and fancy jargon and seek a connection with their audience. In order for you to "connect" with your interviewer, you will need to learn what these effective communicators already know.

General Schwarzkopf returned from the Gulf War in 1991 as a hero and a media star. His briefings during Desert Storm were riveting and dynamic. Upon returning to the United States he gave a speech to the Joint Session of Congress and received a standing ovation. He then gave a speech at West Point, abandoned his notes at the podium, and walked into the audience among the young cadets telling them what skills they needed to succeed in the contemporary army. He received $5 million for his memoirs (the most ever paid for memoirs) and commands $60 thousand per speech.

Why is General Schwarzkopf such a superstar? Is it only because he helped win a war? No. He knows how to communicate, effectively, persuasively, and above all, he's believable. He reaches that part of our mind which reacts to openness, feeling, enthusiasm, and energy—the primitive brain.

USE CHARISMA TO BUILD THE BRIDGE TO CREDIBILITY AND TRUST.

THE EMOTIONAL GATEKEEPER (THE PRIMITIVE BRAIN)

In all of the presidential elections since 1960, those who won reached our primitive brain; those who lost didn't. How can you increase your chances of getting accepted to PA school? By reaching the primitive brain. It is the secret of believability! It's real, physical, and powerful. Neglect it, ignore it, fail to harness its power and you'll likely fail to connect at the interview.

In 1988 Governor Dukakis, in his race for the White House, managed to snatch defeat from the jaws of victory because he failed to connect with the people. In 1984 Walter Mondale did the same thing. Bill Walsh has eluded broadcasting fame because he can't connect. Dan Rather, although the anchor for CBS News, is the reason why CBS lags behind ABC and NBC with respect to network news ratings. These people don't know the secret which I will share with you later.

"But I'm not in the public eye," you might say. As PAs, we're all in the public eye. The ability to communicate effectively is the single most important skill you need to succeed as a PA.

So why do these people miss the boat? They fail to realize that communication is a contact sport.

COMMUNICATION IS A CONTACT SPORT

In 1988 governor Dukakis spent $60 million on his campaign and lost—why? He was ahead by 17 points in the polls after the convention, and just before the debates. Experts said "Dukakis is more knowledgeable than Bush." After the debates, however, although Dukakis won according to the radio audience, Bush was declared the victor largely because of the TV audience. The L.A. *Times* quoted Bush winning 47% to 26%, and CBS had Bush winning 48% to 25%. As we all know, Bush won the election.

It was a similar story with Ronald Reagan versus Mondale in 1984. The Democrat won on radio, but the Republican won with the larger television audience. Bush and Reagan understood what Dukakis and Mondale totally missed; you must make an emotional connection with your audience.

Let's look at Bill Walsh, the renowned ex-professional football coach. He won Super Bowls with the San Francisco 49ers, he is technically precise, experienced, good looking, and considered a football genius. This is the perfect combination for a career as a successful broadcaster, right? The problem is that Bill Walsh has a nasal voice, he rarely smiles, and most of all, he fails to recognize that communication is a contact sport. He went from a short stint in the broadcast booth to coaching college football, and now he's back with the 49ers as a consultant.

In contrast, there's John Madden. He quit as the Oakland Raiders' football coach, he has a face that only a mother could love, and he's extremely difficult to schedule because he won't fly. Yet John Madden has million-dollar contracts with the Fox TV network, Miller Lite, and Ace hardware—why? He has charisma, credibility, and trust. He's honest, natural, likable, and most of all, he's believable.

CREATING EMOTIONAL IMPACT

SELL YOURSELF TO CREATE EMOTIONAL IMPACT

While preparing for one of my seminars, I received an e-mail from a person on the staff of a PA program in the southern United States. He wanted to "join the team" and help us out with our upcoming seminar. I wrote back thanking him for his interest, but telling him that we were not looking to hire anyone at this point. A week later, I received a telephone call from another person wanting to come aboard and help us out. This person, Chris, told me that he had seven years' experience on one of the local PA program's admissions committee. He sold me on the idea that he would truly be an asset to our program. He understood the power of a living résumé versus ink on paper (or a computer screen.) Chris understood that he was selling himself, and we offered him a position. What are you selling?

Some people become uncomfortable when I mention the word "selling." But we all sell ourselves every day. We sell our ideas, our concepts, our reasons why the admissions committee should select us over other highly qualified candidates.

THE SECRET

If you buy into the fact that we are all selling something, then you must understand this crucial point: **The admissions committee selects candidates based on emotion and justifies its decision with facts.** That's the secret I promised to share with you.

After a candidate walks out of the interview room, the committee doesn't sit down with a yellow pad, draw a line down the center, and list the positives and negatives with respect to your presentation. Rather, the decision to accept you or not is more influenced by emotional factors versus rational factors alone. If they like you on an emotional level, they'll justify giving you a higher score by commenting on your GPA, test scores, experience, or whatever will work to support this emotionally based decision. If the committee doesn't like you on an emotional level, you can have a 4.0 gpa, 1300 SAT scores, and 10 years' experience as an inner city EMT, and you still may not win their support.

STATISTICS ARE COLD AND CEREBRAL

In 1960 JFK trailed Nixon at the polls 53% to 47%. By election day, however, JFK shot ahead—why? TV. Nixon won on radio with debating points, but JFK won the television audience on emotion. Nixon tried to appeal based on facts, records, and statistics. "I attended 217 meetings with the National Security Council. I attended 163 cabinet meetings and presided over 19 of them. I visited 54 countries. . . ," etc., etc., etc. The problem is that statistics are cold and cerebral, and so too, the nation concluded, was Richard M. Nixon. The cold-war-weary voters found Kennedy reassuring when compared to Nixon. JFK understood how to make emotional contact with his audience.

Are you what I call a "paper star"? You look great on paper and feel that your GPA and experience alone should get you into PA school. That's not how it works. PAs must communicate on a daily basis with their patients, physicians, and families. If you are too cold and too cerebral, you won't connect in this arena either. This is why any PA program worth its salt will interview candidates, and not select students based on applications alone.

Some people seem to intuitively grasp what it means to communicate effectively and emotionally. The rest of us have to learn it and work at it. This chapter will provide you with all of the techniques that you need to create an emotional connection with others.

These techniques, which will improve your eye contact, energetic delivery, and the ability to think on your feet, to name just a few, will enhance your personal impact in communicating with the admissions committee.

WE ALL SELL OURSELVES EVERY DAY.

THE ADMISSIONS COMMITTEE SELECTS CANDIDATES BASED ON EMOTION AND JUSTIFIES ITS DECISION WITH FACTS.

BEING A "PAPER STAR" IS NOT ENOUGH; YOU MUST BE ABLE TO MAKE AN EMOTIONAL CONNECTION WITH THE COMMITTEE.

THREE TRUTHS

Personal impact is power. Power to achieve whatever you want in your personal life and career. The secret to obtaining personal power is based on three fundamental truths.

Truth # 1:
The spoken word is almost the polar opposite of the written word.

The written word is linear, single channel communication that goes directly to the cerebral cortex, a highly developed reasoning and analytical portion of the brain. The spoken word is multichannel, and includes a kaleidoscope of non-verbal cues such as posture, eye contact, energy, volume, intonation, and much more. Spoken communication carries energy, feeling, passion, and goes directly to the emotional center of the brain—the primitive brain.

The facts are clear: if all you want to do is transfer information, put it in writing. But if you need to motivate, persuade, and influence people, say it with impact.

Truth #2
What you say must be believed in order to have impact.

FOR YOUR MESSAGE TO BE BELIEVED, YOU MUST BE BELIEVED.

No message, regardless of how eloquently stated, brilliantly defended, and painstakingly documented, is able to penetrate a wall of distrust, apprehension, and indifference. For your message to be believed, you must be believed.

We interviewed a young woman who was an accomplished actress. She presented us with a very fancy, and off-beat, résumé. At the bottom right-hand corner of the résumé, below all of her "Off-Broadway" credits, she typed, "Special Talents: I can tie a cherry stem into a knot with my tongue." Although I personally thought this was very funny, she already started to lose her credibility with me before she even walked into the room. Apparently one of my colleagues was even more offended. We asked the applicant to tell us about her most memorable patient and she started to cry. My colleague asked her at this point, "How do we know you're not acting now?" She was stunned. She didn't get in.

Our "gut feeling" on whether we like and believe someone or not is based on emotion versus logic and fact. Does your voice crack? Do your eyes flicker and dart? Is your posture wrong? Do your hands fidget? Are you acting?

Truth #3
Believability is determined at the preconscious level.

Perhaps this is the most important truth. Where does believability come from? You can't build believability out of a mountain of facts and figures. You can't even build it out of a stack of eloquently crafted words. Authoritative credentials, a title, or a letter of recommendation from a "big shot" may give you some credibility and get you to the interview, but you still have to be believable to close the sale, or get accepted to PA school.

These are five rules to make yourself more believable:

1. Make eye contact.
2. Smile.
3. Use open gestures.
4. Use a firm handshake.
5. Have good posture and a strong voice.

INTERVIEWERS ARE BOMBARDED WITH VISUAL STIMULI WHICH REGISTER AT THE PRECONSCIOUS LEVEL

The moment we walk into the interview, we begin giving off a series of verbal and non-verbal cues. Do we walk tall into the room, or do we slump? Do we give a firm handshake, or to we have a wet, limp handshake? Do we refer to our patients as "legs and hearts," or do we refer to them by name? Do we refer to nurses in a derogatory manner, or do we give them the respect they deserve?

An enormous amount of communication is taking place as these thousands of multichannel impressions are carried to your brain. Most of these impressions register at the preconscious level. As a result of these impressions, your brain forms a continuous stream of emotional judgments and assessments. Do I trust this person? Is he or she honest, evasive, friendly, threatening? Is he interesting, boring, warm, cold, anxious? Is she confident, insecure, hiding something?

The emotional judgment that's formed in your preconscious mind about the speaker determines whether you will tune in to his or her message or tune out. If you don't believe in someone at the emotional level, little of what they say will get through.

YOUR BODY LANGUAGE AND VERBIAGE CAN MAKE YOU OR BREAK YOU.

DISCOVERING PRIMITIVE BRAIN POWER

THE $25 MILLION LESSON

In 1989, Deborah Norville was hired by NBC to co-host the *Today* show with Jane Pauley. This was a classic case of "It ain't broke, so we fixed it!" Norville is intelligent and has journalistic credibility, but she also seems unapproachable and cold. Jane Pauley became lost in the shuffle, and in December 1989 a misty-eyed Pauley said goodbye to the *Today* show.

When Pauley left, she took the dynamic chemistry with her. Don't worry about Jane, however; she came back strong. The uncertain future wasn't Jane Pauley's, but the *Today* show itself. With Jane the show enjoyed a 4.4 rating and a 21 share. In the first quarter of 1990 the show dropped to a 3.5 rating and an 18 share. The total cost to NBC was $25 million. Heads rolled and people were fired.

What does Jane Pauley have that Deborah Norville doesn't? In a word, warmth. An open smile with a touch of wit behind it. An honest sense of humor, a delightful sparkle. A bit of the "girl next door" quality. Deborah Norville offers a sexy brand of competence and the cool, unapproachable beauty of a prom queen. NBC seriously miscalculated thinking that Americans would prefer to wake and have breakfast with the prom queen rather than the girl next door.

Eventually, NBC saw the light and hired Katie Couric. Soon after, the ratings soared again—why? She has that "girl next door" quality too. Glamour is not the key ingredient. Beauty and competence are not enough. You must learn to connect with your audience.

HOW DOES THE BRAIN WORK (ANATOMY & PHYSIOLOGY 101)

All communication must pass the gatekeeper: the primitive brain. Will our message get through or be blocked? Do you represent friend or foe? Do you know how to befriend the gatekeeper?

THE PRIMITIVE BRAIN: IT'S REAL, PHYSICAL, AND POWERFUL.

Contrary to what you've probably been taught, effective communication is only partly concerned with our intellectual human brain, or neocortex (new brain). Before we can communicate effectively with our listeners' new brain, we must consider a hidden and generally unrecognized part of ourselves. The primitive brain, although it is hidden from our consciousness, is real, it is physical, and it is extremely powerful.

If the top brass at NBC understood how this worked, Jane Pauley would still be hosting the *Today* show and NBC would be millions richer. If Michael Dukakis understood how the primitive brain works, he might have gone to the White House. It's not mysterious, but it is new. The last ten years have increased our knowledge of the brain ten-fold. We can now analyze why certain people behave in certain ways to make that all-important connection in their communication. We call it "Demystifying Charisma."

Very simply, our brain is composed of the first brain, or primitive brain, and the new brain (neocortex), or cerebral cortex. The cerebral cortex is the thinking, rational portion of our brain. The new brain is 3 to 4 million years old. The left side of our new brain deals with learning, math, and writing. The right side of our new brain deals with art and inspiration. The new brain, however, pales in significance to the primitive, first brain.

The primitive brain is the non-rational, emotional part of our brain: the gatekeeper. The primitive brain is 200 to 500 million years old and is composed mainly of the limbic system. The primitive brain is the seat of human emotion. Your task in the interview is to reach the primitive brain first.

THE GOAL: GET TO THE NEW BRAIN VIA THE PRIMITIVE BRAIN

When people communicate by the spoken word, they almost invariably aim the message at the new brain and completely overlook the primitive brain. That's why even competent and intellectual people such as Michael Dukakis, Deborah Norville, and Bill Walsh fail to effectively communicate their message to their audiences. This is not to say that the new brain is unimportant; on the contrary, our goal is really to get our message to the new brain because that's the decision making part of our brain. But to reach our new brain our message must first pass the primitive brain—the emotional part of the brain. If we ignore this, our message will be distorted or diminished, or it may not get through at all.

It's the listener's primitive brain that decides whether or not to trust you. It's the primitive brain that decides whether a person represents comfort and safety or anxiety and menace. The key to understanding the primitive brain is recognizing that its sole purpose is survival. It quickly analyzes all incoming data and asks the question—Is this situation safe? Friend or foe? You must convince your listener's primitive brain that you are likeable—that you represent warmth, comfort, and safety.

Try this exercise. Take your right hand and make a fist with your right thumb pointing at your face. Now take your left hand, palm facing down, and wrap it around your right fist. This model represents your brain. Your left hand represents your cerebral cortex, the thinking, decision-making portion of the brain. Your right fist is your primitive brain and includes the limbic system. From here arises memory, pain, pleasure, and the ability to balance the extremes of emotion. Now you ask, what is that thumb doing pointing at my face? And here is one of the most important new discoveries, the connection between the sensory organs and the primitive brain. Your right thumbnail represents your eyes. The thumb represents the nerve pathways from your eyes to the primitive brain. All of your sensory input, visual from the eyes, sound from the ears, touch, taste, and smell, goes to the primitive brain **first!**

Now that you understand the physiological relationship between the primitive brain and the new brain from the model of your left hand surrounding your right fist, let's review and examine some of the differences between these two brain systems. The primitive brain is 300 to 500 million years old; the new brain is 3 to 4 million years old. The primitive brain is instinctual and primitive; the new brain is intellectual and advanced. The primitive brain is emotional; the new brain is rational. Most important, perhaps, is that the primitive brain is unconscious and the new brain is conscious.

Today, scientists are rejecting the notion of man being simply a thinking machine, and are beginning to see human beings instead as biological organisms whose survival depends on constant interaction with the environment. Emotions contain the "wisdom of the ages," as one expert put it.

THE LIMBIC SYSTEM

The limbic system, embedded deep in the brain, encompasses all sensory input. For example, have you ever had an immediate and strong emotional response when you first caught the smell of baking bread in the oven, or the scent of fall leaves on a crisp autumn day, or the salt spray of the ocean? Although your new brain will figure out where the feeling comes from, often lodged deep within your memory, it was the olfactory bulbs of the limbic system that gave that emotional reaction even before you became conscious of why. Smell and the sound of music both appear to be the language of the primitive brain, often triggering an immediate emotional response.

When I sold real estate, we were trained to place a teaspoon of vanilla in a small pan in a hot oven before we showed the property. Why? The vanilla gave off the scent of bread. This powerful scent has a strong reaction on the buyers olfactory bulbs which makes them feel like they are in a "home" versus a building.

Scientists now believe that the limbic area is not only the center of emotional stimulus, but it is the main switching station for all sensory input. It determines what sensory input is passed on to the new brain for analysis and decision making, and what input is filtered out and ignored.

Leslie Hart is the brain expert who wrote *How The Brain Works*. He said this about gatekeeping: "Much evidence now indicates that the limbic area in the first brain is the main switch in determining what sensory input will go to the neocortex and what decisions will be accepted from it."

All of the signals that you give off when you speak, including your mannerisms, gestures, eye contact, inflection, and other non-verbal cues, pass through the limbic system for processing. Now if these non-verbal cues convince the limbic system that you are friendly, the message gets a clear channel to the decision-making processes in the new brain. But, if these cues suggest that you are an uncomfortable, threatening presence, the limbic system will alter or block your message.

So if we are energetic, enthusiastic, and believable, our words will actually be given more impact and energy by the listener's primitive brain before they are switched to the new brain. But if we appear boring, anxious, and insecure, our words may not even reach their destination. Instead, our message will be discolored or even tuned out at the switching station by a lack of believability.

EMOTIONS CONTAIN THE WISDOM OF THE AGES.

WHO WE TRUST AND WHY—WE LEARNED AS A BABY.

How, then, do we make friends with the gatekeeper so that our message can get through the gate? How do we become primitive brain friendly? By being natural, by learning to use natural energy, enthusiasm and gestures—all the multichannel, non-verbal cues that enable us to make emotional contact with our listeners. Emotion is the key to making communication memorable. To persuade and achieve your goals, you must understand the primitive brain concept. It all depends on you.

GETTING TO TRUST

How do we use our natural self to reach the primitive brain of our listeners? You've got to be believed to be heard. When dealing with people, trust and believability are synonymous. You can't have one without the other. To communicate effectively with others, you must be trusted. And to win their trust, you must be believable. Belief is a primitive brain function; it's acceptance on faith, it's emotionally based, and it bypasses the intellect. Your primitive brain speaks the language of behavior.

While our new brain sifts our communication for content, data, and facts, our primitive brain sifts for nuances of behavior. Does the voice quiver, or does it project authority? Do your eyes flicker hesitantly or gaze unflinchingly? Is your posture confident or diffident? This is the language of the primitive brain, the language of trust.

Who we trust and why—we learned as a baby. One day my son and I were at the airport in Hartford, Connecticut. We were on our way to Orlando to give a seminar. While sitting in the chairs by our gate, we noticed a toddler come walking over to us with a smile from ear to ear. She was cooing and drooling and having a grand old time. My son and I both played peek-a-boo with her and she giggled happily. Then she walked over to a man with her big smile, and he gave her a very serious look which said "I'm not interested little girl, go away, you bother me." The little girl's face went from a huge smile to a little pout. She then ran from the man knowing instinctively that he represented trouble; he was not safe.

You can't communicate with a baby with words; rather, we must use facial expressions, energy, and sound. The baby responds with the same set of verbal cues. The smile is the language of primitive brain communication. Even a baby knows that a person who doesn't smile lacks warmth and safety. We learn early that the people we should trust are those who smile. To communicate effectively, we must relearn the language of trust.

Did you ever meet someone and instantly like or dislike him or her but you didn't know why? When you meet someone for the first time, your primitive brain receives thousands of non-verbal cues which are registered at the preconscious level. Your intuition comes from this; you form an almost immediate impression of that person. You form an impression that is detailed and often richly colored with emotion.

Most candidates approach the interview as though it's all new brain communication. Their arguments are logic and reason; gpa, test scores, medical experience, etc. The fact is, an equal or greater part of all human communication is primitive brain intuition. When you leave the interview, we say, "I liked him" or "I didn't like her" or "I don't trust him" or "There's something about her that I really like."

Some people can naturally do this without understanding how it works. The candidate who speaks the language of the primitive brain, the language of trust, is the candidate most likely to be believed and accepted. That language communicates very rapidly and effectively.

THE LIKEABILITY FACTOR

In 1984 President Reagan ran for re-election against Walter Mondale. A Gallup Poll looked at three areas with respect to the candidates: issues, party affiliation, and likeability. On the issues, the candidates were considered to be dead even. The Democrat clearly had the edge when it came to party affiliation, however. With respect to likeability, though, Reagan had the edge and won the election. It was the personality factor that dominated.

As applicants, we pride ourselves on a great GPA, our medical experience, and our test scores. But when it's time to interview, it's your likeability that determines whether or not you receive a letter of acceptance or rejection. And as soon as you walk into that interview room, it's the visual connection that sets the beginning of trust and believability.

THE EYE FACTOR

The eye is the only sensory organ that contains brain cells. Memory experts invariably link the objects they remember to a visual image. Research shows that it's the visual image that makes the greatest impact in communication.

The spoken message is made up of only three components:

► The **verbal** component
► The **vocal** component
► The **visual** component

A few years ago, a prominent UCLA professor conducted a landmark study on the relationship of the three components of the spoken word. He measured the effect of each of these three components on the believability of the spoken message. The **verbal** message, or the actual words we use, are what most people mistakenly concentrate on. In fact, this is actually the smallest part of the spoken message. The **vocal** component is made up of the intonation, projection, and resonance of your spoken message. It is the **visual** message, however, the emotion and expression of your body and face as you speak, that carries the most weight.

He also found that the degree of consistency or inconsistency between these three key elements is the factor that determines the believability of your message. The more these three factors harmonize, the more believable you are as a candidate. If your verbal message is not in harmony with your body language, you send a mixed signal to the primitive brain. Your message may or may not get through to the decision-making new brain. The three components of the spoken message are quantified as follows:

► **Verbal** = 7%
► **Voice** = 38%
► **Visual** = 55%

In other words, what you see is what you get. If you come into the interview room yawning, or dressed inappropriately, nothing you do or say will help you. The interviewer's primitive brain has already decided your fate.

> **IT'S YOUR LIKEABILITY THAT DETERMINES WHETHER YOU RECEIVE A LETTER OF ACCEPTANCE OR REJECTION.**

HOW DO WE ENHANCE VERSUS INHIBIT OUR MESSAGE?

The first way we enhance our communication is with eye contact. This is the number one skill to develop; it's primitive brain to primitive brain. The three rules and exercises for maintaining eye contact are as follows:

Rules

1. Use involvement rather than intimacy or intimidation.
2. Count to five (involvement), then look away.
3. Don't dart your eyes; this represents a lack of confidence.

Exercises

1. **Use video feedback.** Tape yourself speaking with someone and watch for your use of, or violation of, the above three rules.
2. **Practice one-on-one.** Have a conversation with someone you trust and ask them for direct feedback with respect to these rules.
3. **Practice with a paper audience.** Place Post-it Notes, with happy faces drawn on them, on a chair and practice counting to five and looking away.

The next way to enhance our message is with posture and movement. A good posture commands attention, and movement shows confidence. Walk into the room standing tall. Don't slump. When you speak to your interviewer, don't be afraid to add movement to your message. You don't have to wave your hands all over the room, but use open gestures to come across as a friendly, open person.

Rules

1. Stand tall.
2. Watch your lower body; don't lean back on one hip or rock back and forth.
3. Get in the ready position; lean slightly forward if you're sitting, or on the balls of your feet if you're standing.
4. Move; show that you're excited, enthusiastic, and confident.

Exercises

1. **Walk away from the wall.** Stand with your back against a wall, heels pressed against the wall along with your head, neck, and shoulders. Try to push the small of your back into the wall. Now simply walk away from the wall and feel how upright and correct your posture is. Try to shake off this posture; you can't. Practice this daily so that when you walk into the interview room, you'll command attention.
2. **Use the ready position.** Remember, if you're standing, sit up slightly on the balls of your feet. If you are sitting, lean slightly forward to your interviewer(s).
3. **Use a paper audience.**

The third way to enhance your message is with dress and appearance. You only get two seconds to make your initial impression on your interviewers. If you blow it, it may take over thirty minutes to recover, and most candidates only get twenty minutes. So it is critical to make a good first impression.

A GOOD POSTURE COMMANDS ATTENTION.

When you are dressed up for an interview, only 10% of your skin is exposed. Please be sure that this 10% is clean, free of extravagant jewelry, shaved, trimmed, combed, and smells good (not overbearing).

Rules

1. Be appropriate; "When in Rome . . ."
2. Be conservative; when in doubt, dress up.
3. Men, always button your jacket.
4. Don't overkill perfume or cologne.
5. Always bring a small mirror and check your face before interviewing.

Exercises

1. **Get people feedback;** ask friends and relatives how well you present yourself.
2. **Be observant; read fashion magazines.** Find a style with which you are comfortable.

The final way to enhance your message is with gestures and your smile. Do you speak with conviction, enthusiasm, and passion? Are you friendly or stuffy? Do you speak with open gestures and a warm smile, or are you a "fig leaf flasher," with your hands always going back and forth covering and uncovering your groin. Remember, openness equals likeability.

Rules

1. Find nervous gestures and stop them.
2. Lift your apples—smile. Make believe you have apples on your cheekbones and try to lift them up to your forehead.
3. Feel your smile.
4. Caution: Phony smiles don't work!

Exercises

1. **Imitate someone who you feel is an effective communicator and play the part with gusto.** Get used to using open gestures and expressions.
2. **Be natural.** Incorporate some of these gestures into your daily communication.

The eye factor rules. The language of the primitive brain is visual language.

THE ENERGY FACTOR

Energy is the fuel that drives the car to success. You don't want to run out of gas when you're halfway up the hill. Think back to the last morning you awoke and felt like you could conquer the world; this was a powerful space to be in. This is where you need to be on interview day—"in the zone," if you will. This next section will focus on ways to unlock your inner energy and present yourself in the best light to the admissions committee.

A. VOICE AND VOCAL VARIETY

Try to use intonation and inflection in your voice. Speaking in a monotone can be deadly and put your listener to sleep. Observe and practice the following rules and exercises to add *pizzazz* to your voice.

Rules

1. Make your voice naturally authoritative; speak from the diaphragm.
2. Put your voice on a roller coaster; practice reading from magazines using intonation and inflection.
3. Be aware of your telephone voice; it represents 84% of the emotional impact when people can't see you.
4. "Smile on the telephone"; people can feel your smile right through the phone.
5. Put your real feelings into your voice.

Exercises

1. **Breathe from the diaphragm.** Take in a deep breath from your nose and let it out slowly, stopping to feel the pressure on your diaphragm. This is where a strong voice originates.
2. **Project your voice.** Try speaking in a normal voice first, then project your voice to reach the back of the room. Try to find the right depth in your voice without straining your vocal chords.
3. **Practice varying your pitch and pace.** Read from magazines.

B. WORDS AND NON-WORDS

Energize with words:

1. Build your vocabulary, especially with synonyms. Instead of "give," use "endow." Instead of "follower," use "disciple." Instead of "cloudy," use "obscure." We provide you with a list of synonyms in the appendix.
2. Paint word pictures. Use motion and emotion with metaphors.
3. Beware of jargon, especially medical jargon. Use "operating room" versus "OR," and "physician" versus "Doc."
4. Avoid meaningless non-words like "ahh," "uhm," "so," "well," "you know," etc. Replace these non-words with a powerful **pause**. A properly timed pause adds drama, energy, and power to your message. Try listening to the famous voice of Paul Harvey if you don't believe me.

C. LISTENER INVOLVEMENT

Humans communicate; books dispense information. Try using these key techniques to add an extra punch to your communication.

1. Use a strong opening. Make it visual and energetic by including pauses, action and motion, and joy and laughter.
2. Maintain eye communication. When you enter the room for a group interview, survey your listeners for 3 to 5 seconds, gauge, and adjust.
3. Lean toward your listeners.
4. Create interest by maintaining eye contact and having high energy.

D. HUMOR

"I will not make age an issue in this campaign. I will not exploit my opponent's youth and inexperience." These words changed the whole campaign for Ronald Reagan when he spoke them at a debate with Walter

A PROPERLY TIMED PAUSE ADDS DRAMA, ENERGY, AND POWER TO YOUR MESSAGE.

Mondale. Reagan knew that he would be asked the "age" question, and he was prepared with a witty response, probably the most remembered thing said at the debate.

We don't recommend that you tell jokes; however, remember, fun is better than funny. The goal is not comedy, but connection. Find the form of humor that works for you, and be natural.

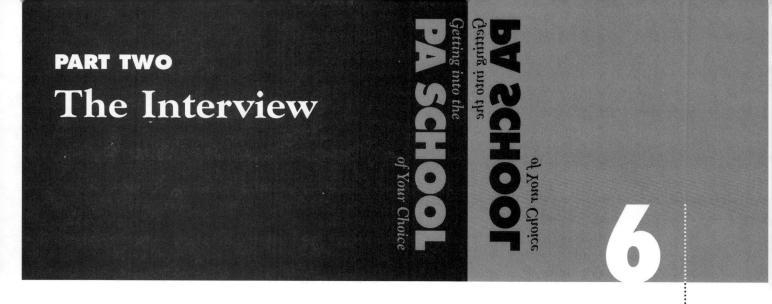

This chapter will cover an overview of the interview process to try and give you a feel of what to expect. In addition, we will provide you with twenty-one tips to help you excel at your interview.

OVERVIEW OF THE INTERVIEW PROCESS

Not all interviews are conducted in the same fashion. The following represents only a sample of what you may face on interview day.

When you get up on the morning of your interview, and before you even get out of bed, ask yourself this question, "What is the worst thing that could possibly happen today?" Once you think about the answer to this question, and accept the fact that you will still have your life, health, and family, you will feel more relaxed and be able to perform to your potential.

Once you arrive at the interview location, someone from the PA program staff will greet you. Whoever that person is, be sure to smile, shake hands, and be polite. You are now officially being evaluated, and this process will continue until you leave in the afternoon or evening.

You will be directed into a room where the other interviewees will be seated (unless you're the first to arrive, of course). Again, you should smile, offer your hand first, and introduce yourself to everyone. Even if someone walks in after you, be the first to extend a handshake and a hello. Remember, you are being evaluated all day, and this is a good way to show off some of your good qualities.

It is a good idea to speak with everyone; ask them about their background, where else they have interviewed, where they are from, etc. Allow others to speak, too. The key is not being too shy or too obnoxious. Find the balance, and, above all, be genuine.

After everyone arrives, you will begin a short series of talks with the Director of the program, the Director of Admissions, and the Financial Aid Officer. Listen intently, ask intelligent questions, and stay relaxed. Do not feel that you have to dominate the situation; you'll have time to shine when the actual interviews start.

Next comes the case scenarios. These are a set of three to four written questions that you will all have about fifteen minutes to answer. They are not meant to stress you out before the interview, but are simply a way to get an idea of your ability to reason and make sound judgments.

BE FRIENDLY AND OUTGOING,
BUT NOT OVERBEARING
OR COCKY.

Once you've finished the case scenarios, you'll be split up into two groups; half of you will begin the interview process, and half of you will attend a class with the first-year students. When you go to the class, remember that you are always being evaluated. Inappropriate comments to students can ruin your day. Pay attention to the lecture, remember the instructor's name, and only ask sensible, relevant questions if you feel it is absolutely necessary. If you like, you may ask the students questions before and after the class.

At most programs, the interviews consist of three parts: the student interview, the group interview, and the single interview. There are usually two students, a first year and a second year. The group interview consists of three PAs or MDs, and the single interviewer is usually the senior PA or a psychologist/psychiatrist. **Please keep in mind that not all programs follow the same interview patterns or procedures.**

After the morning interviews, you will have lunch, meet with some of the current students, and then switch roles with the other applicants. If you already interviewed, do not make any comments about the questions or process.

At the end of the day you will all be offered a tour of the facility. We recommend that you take this tour unless you have a flight or train to catch. If that's the case, let the Dean know that you have to keep to your schedule, and thank her for the opportunity to interview. If you go on the tour, ask intelligent questions, don't fool around, and most importantly, ask yourself if this is the kind of place where you'd like to go to school.

THE STUDENT INTERVIEW

Although this tends to be the most relaxed interview, let your guard down and you could find yourself reapplying next year. The students take this interview very seriously, and they could make you or break you. They usually do not have access to all of your application, but they will score you and comment on your performance. They basically want to know three things about you:

1. Do you know what a PA is and does?
2. Have you worked as hard as they have to get here?
3. Would you make a good classmate?

Keep in mind that students tend to grade tougher than the other committee members. Remember in grade school when the teacher allowed the students to grade their own papers; we're much tougher on ourselves. Students have a great sense of pride in their accomplishments, their school, and the PA profession. Don't blow it by making comments like, "You're only students" or "The hard part is over; you guys will be easy." You might as well say goodbye now.

A good tip is to ask the students what they like about the program and why they like it. Ask them why you should pick this school, if given the opportunity, over Duke, or Yale, or Emory, for example. Let them sell you a little bit.

NOT ALL PROGRAMS FOLLOW THE SAME INTERVIEW PATTERNS OR PROCEDURES.

LET YOUR GUARD DOWN WITH THE STUDENTS AND YOU WILL FIND YOURSELF REAPPLYING NEXT YEAR.

THE GROUP INTERVIEW

For some, this is the toughest part of the day. I've seen applicants cry, get mad, clam up, shake, rattle, and roll in this interview. In this one you usually have three or more committee members, usually PAs and MDs, who have just re-read your application and have specific, and general, questions in mind. The committee has six basic things to find out from you:

1. Do you have a good concept of the PA profession?
2. Can you handle the program academically?
3. Will you "fit in" with the class, and will you be able to contribute to it?
4. Are you a compassionate person?
5. Are you a team player?
6. Can you handle the stress of the program?

It is your job to convince the group that the answer is yes on all accounts. We will cover the questions, and specific answers, in the next chapter.

The group has no hidden agenda; they're really not trying to trip you up. Some applicants become very defensive when asked certain questions. Remain cool, never raise your voice, and, as the commercial says, "Never let them see you sweat." The committee wants you to do well; some of these people may have even originally scored your application to get you here.

The following are some general tips for interviewing:

► Be honest
► Be genuine
► If you don't know the answer, admit it
► Don't beg to be accepted
► Think! Think! Think!
► Smile
► Make eye contact

Once the committee interview is over, you'll be asked if you have any questions. See the end of the chapter for a short list of appropriate questions to ask the committee. You do not have to ask questions. In fact, the committee will not care one way or the other if you ask questions or not. The exception is asking too many questions at the interview, or asking inappropriate questions.

Before you leave the room, be sure to thank each member of the group by name.

THE INDIVIDUAL INTERVIEW

The purpose of this interview is threefold:

1. To verify what you have told the other interviewers.
2. To see if your answers are consistent.
3. To find out more about your personal life.

Please be consistent with your answers. If you have done your homework, you'll have no problem. For instance, don't think that you can tell

> REMEMBER: ALL OF THE INTERVIEWERS WANT YOU TO DO WELL; NOBODY WANTS TO TRIP YOU UP.

> BE CONSISTENT WITH YOUR ANSWERS.

the students and the group interviewers that you never thought of going to medical school, and then confide in the single interviewer that you applied twice but weren't accepted. This is inconsistent and may lower your score.

If you draw a psychologist for your single interviewer, he/she may ask you very personal questions. Don't get flustered. Don't volunteer too much information, either. Avoid talking about drugs, sexual preference, the family alcoholic, and topics which may get you into trouble. If they hand you a rope, don't hang yourself.

SCORING/RATING YOUR INTERVIEW

THESE SIX AREAS MAY BEST SUMMARIZE THE QUALITIES OF A GOOD PA.

After each interview session, morning and afternoon, the entire committee meets to discuss the candidates, compare notes, and give you a score. You may be rated in six areas; within these, each committee may decide on common indicators which best summarize the qualities of a good PA.

1. Cognitive/Verbal Ability

The committee wants to know if you have the ability to think through a problem and respond appropriately. Are you a life-long learner? Can you articulate your ideas clearly and succinctly? Do you present your ideas in a logical sequence? How perceptive are you about others? Here, both verbal ability and written skills are important indicators. The committee will also want to see evidence of your organizational skills, for instance, time-management strategies, or your ability to prioritize, and indeed problem-solving processes. You need to show too that you understand the rigor of the PA program of study.

2. Motivation to Become a PA

Are you strongly motivated or just testing the water? Why do you want to become a PA? Are you interested in patients or the science of medicine? The committee will want to get a sense of your enthusiasm and commitment to the profession. You will need to demonstrate that you are a practical person who has had experience with patient care.

3. Understanding of the PA Profession

Do you know what PA practice entails? Do you know any PAs? Have you worked with any PAs? In this area, the committee will be looking to see if you are realistic in your understanding of the role of a PA and that you also have a positive attitude towards RNs/MDs. Once again, the committee will be interested to see how patient oriented you are.

4. Interpersonal Skills/Behavior

Do you work collaboratively? Would you be respected by patients and colleagues? Or do you come across as too eager and domineering? Are you courteous and tactful in dealing with others? Are you compassionate? There are a range of key areas within this category, from good grooming and personal presentation to more complex communication skills where the panel will be looking to see that you demonstrate appropriate listening skills, have an understanding of different audiences, are warm and open without being overly friendly, and can be diplomatic when required. Obviously, coming across as too aggressive or fabricating your experience to win points are not indicators a panel would want to find.

5. Ability to Handle Stress

Except for a little anxiety, can you relax and be at ease? Do you have a sense of humor? Are you articulate? Do you convey your ideas clearly? Do you remain poised and relatively calm in the face of stressful situations? Do you remain self-confident without being over-confident or cocky? Do you have a measure of self-possession? Are you over-anxious or confused in times of stress?

6. Personal Characteristics

Are you thoughtful and innovative? Are you a technician or a decision maker? Are the facts you present in your interview consistent with your written file? Some of the key areas that a panel may look for here are your level of maturity, self-drive, and determination, balanced with how flexible and creative you may be. Your ability to empathize with others will also be an important indicator in this area.

Each program has its own rating system. For instance, a scale of 1–10 may be used, with 10 being the best (accept) and 1 being the worst (reject); or a scale which places applicants in one of the following categories—Definite Acceptance, Probable Acceptance, Uncertain, Probable Rejection, Definite Rejection. After each session of interviews is over, the committee meets in one room to give the final scores. An applicant's name will be called, and each committee member will simply call out his or her score. Once the scores are collected on all of the applicants, the discussions begin. **Again, each program has its own method of evaluating interviewees.**

If an applicant scores all 1's or all 10's, there's nothing to discuss. Most applicants, however, fall somewhere in the middle and require further discussion. For instance, if the students score an applicant 10 and 10, respectively; the group scores the applicant 10, 8, and 10, respectively; and the single interviewer scores the same applicant a 4, there's obviously a problem here. What does the single interviewer know that the rest of the committee doesn't?

Upon asking the single interviewer, we may find out that everything went well until the applicant mentioned his problem with drugs and alcohol. This is a problem. At this point, the students and group change their scores and the applicant does not get in.

The process can also work in reverse. Someone may really champion an applicant and convince everyone else to give a better score. There are an extensive number of checks and balances set up to be sure that only the best candidates get accepted.

INTERVIEWING TIPS/RULES

1. Arrive to the interview on time.
2. Dress appropriately.
   Men: suit and tie
   Women: business suit
   Shined shoes
3. Bring a compact mirror to check for "crumbs."
4. Smile genuinely.
5. Always offer your (firm) handshake first.
6. Look everyone in the eyes.

EACH PROGRAM HAS ITS OWN RATING SYSTEM AND USES ITS OWN EVALUATION CRITERIA.

7. Speak clearly and loud enough to be heard.
8. Use proper English.
9. Say "please" and "thank you."
10. Don't sit until asked to do so.
11. Bring a copy of your entire application; review it when you have time.
12. Have a short number of good questions to ask.
13. Bring a picture of yourself.
14. When interviewing, try not to make nervous hand movements.
15. Don't become defensive.
16. Don't ever raise your voice.
17. Don't say too much.
18. Speak to everyone with genuine interest.
19. Be consistent.
20. Answer the question briefly.
21. Don't ramble.

GOOD QUESTIONS TO ASK

YOU ARE NOT OBLIGATED TO ASK QUESTIONS AT THE END OF THE INTERVIEW.

After you finish each interview, you will be given the opportunity to ask questions. You do not have to ask any questions, and if you don't, it won't be counted against you. But, if you ask inappropriate questions, or too many questions, you're liable to annoy the interviewer(s). If you choose not to ask any questions, simply say, "No thank you, I've had all of my questions answered already." If you do ask questions, use the following list as a guide:

Ask Students

▶ What do you like best about this program?
▶ Why should I pick this program over any other program?
▶ What do you like least about this program?

Ask the Group

▶ If I'm selected, why should I pick this program over Duke or GW?
▶ What is this school's **first-time** pass/fail rate on the national boards?
▶ What is the highlight of this program?

Ask the Single Interviewer

▶ Why is this program so successful?
▶ What can be improved about this program?
▶ What is this school's **first-time** pass/fail rate on the boards? *

Do Not Ask

DO NOT ASK INAPPROPRIATE QUESTIONS.

▶ So, what do you do for excitement?
▶ How's the partying around here?
▶ Are there lots of women/men here?

These are inappropriate questions to ask of an interviewer.

*You'll notice that we ask this question twice; that's how important it is to know. It also shows some consistency, and it is a very good question to ask.

AFTER THE INTERVIEW

After you go home from the interview, write a letter of thanks to the Director of the program. This will be placed in your file, whether you get in or not, and if it's the latter, it may help you next year.

The Interview

In our last chapter we focused on the interview process and the particular skills you must exhibit to perform well. In this chapter we will focus on the exact questions that you are likely to be asked, and provide you with an insider's slant on what they **really** want to know.

Too many applicants feel that they can come to the interview and just "wing it." This can be a fatal mistake. In this climate of hundreds of applicants for too few slots, you must practice, practice, practice. If you don't, you may find yourself applying again next year.

We do not recommend that you memorize the exact answers to the questions we give here. This too can be a fatal mistake. Rather, we encourage you to incorporate the concept into your own experiences and formulate an answer that is specific to you and your situation.

The questions and answers will be set up in this format:

► Question:
► In other words:
► Answer:

We will first give you the question. Then we will tell you what the question really asks for. Finally, we will give an appropriate response. The first six areas will cover those discussed in the last chapter—scoring/rating the interview. The remainder are more questions that you could very likely be asked. Keep your answers short but concise.

COGNITIVE/VERBAL ABILITY

Question: How has your academic work prepared you for the PA profession?

In other words: Can you handle the rigor of our didactic phase?

Answer: If you have filled out your work sheets from Chapter 5, you will be well prepared to answer this one. "I have a B.S. in chemistry with a 3.3 GPA. In addition, I recently completed a Microbiology course and Anatomy and Physiology, receiving an A in each class. Throughout college, I worked at a part-time job and volunteered at the local hospital."

DO NOT COME TO THE INTERVIEW WITH THE INTENTION OF "WINGING IT."

INCORPORATE YOUR OWN ANSWERS TO THESE QUESTIONS.

This applicant not only demonstrates the ability to handle difficult science course work; she also demonstrates good time management skills and the ability to do more than one thing at a given time.

Question: Tell us about the last book you read.

In other words: Tell us something about yourself—your interests.

Answer: You don't want to mention that you read the last Danielle Steele novel. Play it safe: "I just read the autobiography of Abraham Lincoln. He surmounted incredible odds to become the President. It is a very inspiring story."

Question: What is the most important issue facing the health care system in the United States?

In other words: Can you articulate an intelligent response to an area that affects all of us as citizens and as health care workers?

Answer: Read the journals recommended throughout this text. When reading the newspaper, focus on these issues which are written about every day. Talk to other PAs and get a sense for what's going on in this arena. How does it affect them?

"I feel that 'managed care' is an important concern at this time. Some providers feel that the insurance companies are now dictating how long a patient can remain in the hospital for a given illness. For example, until recently, mothers were allowed only one day in the hospital after having a baby, so-called "drive-by" deliveries. On the other hand, however, we must do something with respect to excessive health care costs. It's a real dilemma."

MOTIVATION FOR A PA CAREER

Question: Why do you want to be a PA?

In other words: Have you thought about this intelligently?

Answer: You must answer this question in 250 words or less and provide an answer which shows insight and enthusiasm.

"After serving as a hospital corpsman for four years and an emergency room technician for one year, I realized that I found a niche in health care. I enjoy providing comfort to patients and placing them at ease. I also enjoy being a member of the team and doing my part to provide the best quality of care to the patient.

I want to do more, however. I would like to be able to diagnose and treat patients as well. Although I love my current job, I feel that I could contribute much more in this newly enhanced role as a PA.

I have thought about medical school; however, I have a family and I do not have the time, nor the inclination, to spend the next eight or so years of my life pursuing that goal. From what I have experienced, PAs have a challenging and rewarding role in the health care system. I have never met a PA who disliked his/her job.

I simply want to practice medicine. I rather like the fact that PAs have physicians available for consultation with difficult presentations. I feel no need to be independent, although I think in situations I'll be somewhat autonomous. This is why I prefer becoming a PA rather than a nurse practitioner, who frequently practices independently.

ANSWER IN 250 WORDS OR LESS.

Finally, I like the fact that PAs are trained in the medical model, in contrast to nursing, and they can move from one specialty to the next without having to re-train. This is a benefit not even afforded the MD."

In less than 250 words, the applicant has managed to answer several questions here and touched on several key points:

► Demonstrates experience
► Teamwork
► Enthusiasm
► Why not MD?
► Why not nurse practitioner?
► Why not nurse?
► Understands dependent practitioner role
► Realizes may still be autonomous

Question: Have you applied to other programs?

In other words: 1) How serious are you? 2) What's your logic in choosing the programs you have?

Answer: By applying to other programs, you show that you want to become a PA and you are maximizing your chances of getting into school. In addition, you should be prepared to discuss why you selected the programs you have.

"I applied to Northeastern, Quinnipiac, and Duke because they offer a Master's degree."

"I applied to Yale, Quinnipiac, Northeastern, and Springfield College because my wife will be supporting me and our children, and, if we have to move, she may not be able to find a job which pays enough to cover the rent and put food on the table."

"I applied to Cornell, Alabama, and Cuyahoga because I'm really interested in doing surgery."

(Note: Your transcripts from the various colleges frequently list the other programs you've applied to. So, many times the committee knows where else you've applied.)

Question: What have you done to prepare yourself for this profession?

In other words: Are you a serious applicant or just testing the water because you're not happy with your current profession?

Answer: Review your worksheets and list all of your preparation and accomplishments to get you here today.

"In addition to my degree in biology, I also worked as a nurse's aide for three years. Recently, I went back to night school to take courses in Cell Biology and Pharmacology. In addition, I have volunteered at the local hospital's HIV clinic for the past 6 months.

I have also shadowed two PAs this year; one works in internal medicine and the other works in OB-GYN. And, I have joined the AAPA and ConnAPA to keep up with current issues facing the profession."

Don't fabricate here. Hopefully, you have done something to prepare yourself for getting into PA school.

WHAT IS YOUR LOGIC FOR APPLYING TO THE PROGRAMS YOU HAVE?

WHY SHOULD THE COMMITTEE SELECT YOU OVER THE 600 OR SO OTHER APPLICANTS?

Question: Have you done anything to increase your chances of being accepted to the PA program?

In other words: This is especially important for re-applicants. Just how serious and committed are you? What makes you stand out from the person sitting next to you this morning?

Answer: This is your opportunity to shine. Tell the committee about all of the PAs you have contacted, shadowed, and communicated with. Tell them about the recent courses you've completed and all of your health care experience. Point out that you have joined your state Academy of Physician Assistants and the American Academy of Physician Assistants. Let them know, by name, any and all of their current students that you have worked with. In other words, demonstrate that getting into PA school has been your mission for the past twelve months.

UNDERSTANDING OF PA PROFESSION

Question: What is your understanding of what PAs do?

In other words: Are you aware of the PA concept?

Answer: Do not recite the AAPA definition of a PA here. Personalize your answer based on your experience with PAs. If you have no experience with PAs, then don't try to fool the committee into thinking you do; you'll be caught. You may want to start like this: "From my understanding . . ."; otherwise, give your understanding of the profession based on first-hand knowledge:

"Based on my experience as a technician in the emergency room, and through my recent shadowing of two PAs, I have observed several PAs in action. Most of them work autonomously but usually have the availability of a physician when needed. In the ER the PAs are usually the first to see the patients when they arrive. They take a short history from the patient or EMTs, perform a physical exam, and order the appropriate tests. At times, they suture, apply casts, or perform various other procedures.

The Internal Medicine PAs are part of a team, working more closely with other students, interns, residents, and the attending physician. They often round with the team and present and discuss their patients. They also report to the ER to interview their patients, write the H&P, order the appropriate tests, and formulate the initial plan."

This applicant is explaining, from personal experience, the role of the PA at her institution. This is much better than giving a definition of the profession, and, believe me, many people will simply cite the definition.

DO YOU HAVE A FIRM GRASP OF THE PA'S ROLE IN HEALTH CARE?

Question: Tell us about the role you see the PA playing in the health care system?

In other words: Are you familiar with the PA concept?

Answer: This is similar to the above question but with a little twist. Do not mention a hierarchy here of physician, PA, nurse, etc. Keep the focus on teamwork.

"PAs are a part of the health care team, working with physicians, nurses, and other members to provide the best care to the patient."

Question: How do you feel about taking call or working 60 or more hours per week as a second-year student?

In other words: Do you know what you're getting yourself into?

Answer: You may be asking about now, "But I thought PAs didn't have to work like interns, putting in so many hours?" While you may choose not to work so many hours as a PA, when you are a PA student and on rotation, you are expected to work as many hours as the medical student or intern. The correct response would be:

"I'm prepared to do whatever it takes to be a PA. I have spoken with several PA students, and I know what I am up against. I welcome the challenge of learning all that I can while I'm in school."

INTERPERSONAL SKILLS/BEHAVIOR

Question: Describe an interaction you have had with a patient which made an impact on you.

In other words: Do you have compassion or are you simply science oriented—more interested in the pathology versus the patient?

Answer: Be prepared to discuss a patient who has made an impact on you in some way. Let the committee know what the situation was, how the patient made out, and what you've learned from him/her.

"My first trauma patient was a 23-year-old Portuguese gentleman who was involved in an industrial fire. He spoke no English. I remember the burn team coming to the ER and assessing him. He appeared to be in no pain, even though he was burned over most of his body. I originally thought he was wearing gloves, until someone pointed out that was his skin hanging from his hands.

The burn team assessed the patient, left the room, and began drawing figures on a piece of paper. They concluded that the man had less than a 3% chance of surviving. They went back into the trauma room, this time with an interpreter, and explained the situation to the patient. They asked him if he wanted them to operate, which would be extremely painful, or simply make him comfortable. I remember his response was to operate. What else would a 23-year-old say, I thought?

The patient died after surgery, but I will never forget him, and how he must have felt lying on the trauma room table, not understanding English, and having someone ask if he preferred to live in pain or die?"

Question: What do you think is the most difficult situation described in the interview scenarios that you completed earlier today? Why?

In other words: Do you have any hidden feelings about AIDS patients, psychiatric patients, or drug addicts?

Answer: Don't shoot yourself in the foot. Hopefully, you did not give any controversial answers, as suggested. You can simply reply, in response to the trauma patient with HIV:

"Every day I witness staff members in the hospital not taking precautions by wearing gloves or protective eyewear. I do my best to lead by example and always protect myself, but I must admit that I cringe when I see others take universal precautions so lightly."

ARE YOU PATIENT ORIENTED OR ARE YOU MORE INTERESTED IN THE SCIENCE OF MEDICINE?

What this applicant has done is to shift the focus off the HIV-positive patient and concentrate on the issue of universal precautions.

ABILITY TO HANDLE STRESS

Question: Describe the most stressful work or academic situation you have been in, and tell us how you dealt with it.

In other words: What constitutes stress to you, and do you know how to cope with stress?

Answer: The committee knows that interviewing for PA school is stress enough, and they probably have a good idea of your ability to handle it at this point. But give them a little more insight by example:

"I find the best way to deal with stress is to avoid it! But we all know that isn't always possible. My most stressful situation came as a junior officer in the Air Force. I was placed in charge of a bomb clean-up operation at Nellis air force base in Nevada. I had forty people working for me—carpenters, explosive ordnance disposal people, and several truck drivers and carpenters. The range we were cleaning was used by F-16 pilots to practice bombing skills. We had to sweep the range, remove the live ordnance which remained, and build new targets. Under each old piece of plywood we found a rattlesnake. Between the bombs and the snakes, I was never so scared in my life; and I was in charge!

To get through this situation, I relied on the senior noncommissioned officers from each group. Each morning we'd meet and make a plan of action. We kept in contact via radio all day. I'm proud to say that we had no casualties, and we all received a letter of accommodation from our commanding officer. Teamwork got us through."

Although this is a dramatic story, for which most of us have no similar experience, the applicant explained that he relied on others' help to get everyone through the situation. He used teamwork and planning each day to get through.

By the way, providing a copy of the letter of accommodation in your application will provide verification for your statement.

Question: How do you usually deal with stress?

In other words: Do you have any stress-relieving activities? Some interviewers may also ask this question to see if you exercise.

Answer: We recommend that you take up some form of exercise for your own good. Then you can answer:

"I run three miles a day."

Question: What kind of personal stress do you see associated with our PA program?

In other words: Do you have a realistic view of the rigor of the program? Do you have any hidden fears about coming here to school?

Answer: After speaking to several of your students, both first year and second year, I am aware of how difficult the two years will be. For instance, I know that the didactic phase is extremely comprehensive

THE BEST WAY TO DEAL WITH STRESS IS TO PREVENT IT!

and fast paced. In addition, I'm aware of the amount of hours I'll be expected to put in on clinical rotations. However, I am confident that my previous college work in chemistry and biology have prepared me well for further study, and I was never afraid to roll up my sleeves and work long, hard hours. I look forward to the challenge."

Question: What kind of stress do you see associated with the PA profession?

In other words: Are you aware of how far the profession has come and what challenges we still have ahead?

Answer: "The PA profession has come a long way in a short time. I know that the early PAs have had to fight for all of the respect and privileges that everyone enjoys today. On the other hand, there are still issues to be resolved and more work to be done. Some nurses and nurse practitioners take issue with the scope of PA practice; a case in point is in Mississippi. We will always face new challenges, especially with health care reform, but the profession has come too far, and if PAs continue doing as well as they have done in the past, the profession will continue to grow."

PERSONAL CHARACTERISTICS

Question: What do you do outside of your work or academic studies?

In other words: Are you a well-rounded person?

Answer: Go back to your work sheets and make a list of your extracurricular activities. List things you like to do: biking, hiking, running, investing, playing in a band, etc.

Question: Please discuss your answer for question #___ on the interview questionnaire? Or, what did you mean by___ on your essay?

In other words: Can you think on your feet?

Answer: As mentioned already, the best way to deal with stress is to avoid it; don't write anything controversial on your questionnaire or narrative, and you'll never have to answer a question like this. But if you do, keep your cool, take a deep breath, and answer the question to the best of your ability. Don't add injury to insult by arguing your point. Perhaps you misunderstood the original question.

Question: Your file indicates that you have had difficulty with ___ (e.g., time management or science course work). Would you like to explain this?

In other words: Have you thought about your shortcomings? What have you done to change things?

Answer: Of course, you would like to comment. You have hopefully anticipated this question about your grades in high school, or why you flunked freshman chemistry in college.

"In high school I had no real focus in life and I simply wanted to graduate. After working for Dr. Smith and realizing I loved medicine, I went to college with a purpose, to get into PA school, and my grades improved tremendously."

Question: What accommodations, if any, do you need to successfully complete the program?

ARE YOU A WELL-ROUNDED PERSON; DO YOU HAVE A LIFE?

In other words: Is there any part of our program that you will not participate in?

Answer: We had several women in our class who weren't thrilled with the idea of classmates doing breast exams on one another. This issue came up at the beginning of our physical exam sessions. It caused a lot of stress for the class and the students involved. If you feel strongly about an issue, with respect to the program, discuss it before you begin the program, but not necessarily at the interview.

MORE INTERVIEW QUESTIONS

The following questions may or may not be similar to the above. Keep in mind that specific examples and vignettes make for better answers than a simple yes or no. By the same token, keep your answers very brief, but concise.

Question: So, tell us a little about yourself?

In other words: Why are you here?

Answer: Dig out those worksheets and compile a brief summary of your accomplishments. In 250 words or less, cover the following points:

1. Your strongest skills
2. Specific areas of knowledge
3. Greatest personality strengths
4. What you do best
5. Key accomplishment

(Note: All of your answers do not have to be medically oriented.)

Question: You have had several jobs in the past; how do we know you will finish the program if we accept you?

In other words: Do you have commitment and staying power?

Answer: This should be a two-part answer:

1. Admit to having moved around a bit. (It's obvious from your application.)
2. Convince the committee that you've "seen the light," if you will, and tell them what specific steps you've taken to achieve your goal.

Question: Why do you think Duke turned you down?

In other words: Did you take the time to find out why they didn't accept you?

Answer: If you interviewed elsewhere, or if you've been turned down for any reason, be sure to follow up on how you can improve your application. The program will usually tell you why you came up short this time.

"I was told that, although I was a good applicant, the pool was so competitive this year, not all good candidates could feasibly be accepted. They told me to continue with my current medical experience."

Question: What are your strengths as an applicant?

In other words: Convince us that you are our woman/man.

HAVE AN IDEA AS TO WHY OTHER PROGRAMS TURNED YOU DOWN.

Answer: We've already answered a similar question above. Be sure to toot your own horn without being too cocky. Review your worksheets for all of the information you'll need on this one.

Question: What are your biggest weaknesses as an applicant, and what do you plan to do to correct them?

In other words: Please tell us that you don't "walk on water" too.

Answer: They may be handing you a rope here, but you don't have to hang yourself. Everyone has weaknesses, but for an interview, you want to stay focused on the positive. Achieve a compromise:

"I tend to work too many hours lately, but I realize how important my free time is and I'm much happier when I get to do the things I love outside of work."

Question: Do you manage your time well?

In other words: Can you handle a program as difficult as this? Will you require constant help?

Answer: "Yes, I do. I have a set of written goals, and I prioritize my time so as to accomplish them all in the order of their importance, and in a timely manner."

(I told you having written goals is important.)

Question: Do you prefer to work with others or by yourself?

In other words: Are you a team player?

Answer: "I prefer to work on a team. However, if necessary, I can work just as well autonomously."

Question: How do you get along with your co-workers?

In other words: Will you make a good classmate?

Answer: "I get along very well with others. I usually reach out to people, or I can simply hold your hand and be a friend in time of need. I consider myself to be a team player."

Question: Your supervising MD tells you to do something that you know is dead wrong; what do you do?

In other words: How's your judgment?

Answer: "I certainly do not know what it is like to be a PA in that situation, but it seems that I would have to bring the possible error to his/her attention, tactfully, and be sure that it gets resolved."

(A little humility goes a long way.)

Question: What interests you most about our school?

In other words: Have you done your homework?

Answer: This is a very personal choice; just be prepared for the question and answer it to the best of your ability. Let the committee know that you have specific reasons for being interested in their school.

Question: What would be your ideal job as a PA?

In other words: Are you open minded?

Answer: The key here is to show that you have an open mind, yet don't try to deceive the committee. If all of your experience is in orthopedics, don't try to tell the committee that you've always wanted to work in an HIV clinic. Give a well-balanced answer:

IF THEY HAND YOU A ROPE, DON'T HANG YOURSELF.

ARE YOU A TEAM PLAYER? WILL YOU MAKE A GOOD CLASSMATE?

DO YOUR HOMEWORK: LEARN ABOUT THE PROGRAMS YOU APPLY TO.

"Although I feel my current interest is in orthopedics, I have never worked in any other area. I know from talking with several of your graduate students that they came into the program with certain inclinations, but after doing a rotation in another specialty liked it enough to work in that area after graduation. I will try to keep an open mind."

Question: What did you learn from your overseas internship/experience?

In other words: What did you learn from your overseas internship/experience?

Answer: That's right, this question is as straightforward as they come, yet too many applicants blow it. Think about your travel overseas, and be prepared to discuss the impact it had on you. Did you take advantage of the local culture? Did you mix with the natives? Did you make any lasting friendships? You didn't blow this opportunity, did you?

Question: What do you want to be doing five years from now?

In other words: Do you have any goals?

Answer: Of course, you do. I won't comment much more here other to say that I hope you still want to be a PA in five years, and that you still want to contribute to the medical community in a positive way.

(Note: If you haven't filled out your goal sheet yet, please do so now.)

Question: Have you ever seen anyone die?

In other words: Are you prepared to deal with death?

Answer: This was a favorite question of one of our committee members, usually before the applicant sat down. If you have never seen anyone die, that's ok. You are not expected to know what it is like to be a PA. If you have seen someone die, reflect on the situation with solitude and explain that you are capable of carrying on. "Death is a part of life."

Don't answer, as one person did, "Of course, I've seen people die. I was in a gang."

INNOCENT QUESTIONS?

There are no innocent questions. Remember, you are being evaluated from the time you walk into the building until the time you get into your car.

Question: How are you today?

In other words: Are you a positive or negative person?

Answer: "I'm fine, thank you." That's all that is required. Do not go on about the parking lot being full, or the terrible night's sleep you had, or how nervous you are.

Question: Did you have any trouble finding us?

In other words: Did you use the resources available to you?

Answer: "No trouble at all; I called the office ahead of time and got great directions from Betty."

Question: What was the last movie you saw?

In other words: What are you interested in?

Answer: We can't tell you what kind of movies to go see. Personally, your author is into horror movies, but I wouldn't tell the admission's committee that. An Oscar winner is always a safe bet.

Question: What was the most difficult question they asked you at Bowman Gray?

In other words: Have you thought about that interview?

Answer: For some reason this question draws the most tears out of applicants. One applicant burst into tears and to the surprise of the interview panel said, "My mother." She was obviously emotionally distraught. Try not to get too emotional at the interview, the committee may take this as being a sign of weakness. Tell the committee that you were well prepared for the interview, and they did not ask you any questions that you did not anticipate.

CLOSING THE INTERVIEW

Question: What will you do if you don't get in this year?

In other words: Will you give up?

Answer: We cover specific steps to take in the next chapter, if you do not get in this year. Do not read too much into this question. They ask this to everyone and want to know if you will apply again.

"I will consult with the program, find out why I was not accepted, and strive to accomplish those things for next year."

Question: Do you have any questions for us?

(We discuss this question and the answer to it in the previous chapter.)

Finally, it is worth repeating that you do not use these same answers at the interview. Study your worksheets, and spend some time compiling your own answers to these questions. Be honest and genuine.

Remember, what's the worst thing that can happen?

BE HONEST AND GENUINE.

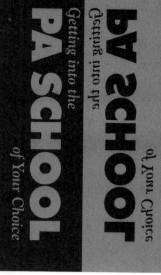

Financial Aid

THE ALL-IMPORTANT QUESTION

Can I afford to go to PA school? The question you should be asking is, can I afford not to go to PA school? If your goal is to become a PA, then the answer to this question is easy. The worst thing you could do is shy away from applying because you think you won't be able to afford it, then live the rest of your life wondering, "what if?"

When I applied to Yale and spoke to students at the open house, they told me that if I got accepted the program would do its best to ensure I got through financially. They were right. I may have borrowed a little more than I intended, but the money was available. As you will soon find out, there are plenty of opportunities for loans, grants, scholarships, etc. It does, however, take a little work on your part. But since you have set your goals and you're focused, you are prepared for anything.

The following chapter is not meant to be a step-by-step guide for filling out financial aid forms. The focus of this book, remember, is getting into the PA school of your choice. The purpose of this chapter is to give you some valuable resources and advice on getting financial aid.

INDIVIDUAL SCHOOL COSTS (at time of writing)

Surgeon's Assistant Program University of Alabama at Birmingham	In State: $6,160 for 24 mos. Out of State: $12,320 for 24 mos.
Charles R. Drew University of Medicine and Science Los Angeles, CA	In State: $10,100 for 24 mos. Certificate: $9,200 for 24 mos. Out of State: same
College of Osteopathic Medicine of the Pacific Pomona, CA	In State: $9,470 for 24 mos. Out of State: same
University of California, Davis Sacramento, CA	In State: $1,527 for 18 mos.; $1,100 for summer quarter Out of State: $2,566 for 18 mos.; $1,100 for summer quarter

Stanford University Palo Alto, CA	In State: $8,300 for 15 mos. Out of State: $13,400 for 15 mos.
University of Southern California School of Medicine Los Angeles, CA	In State: $38,000 for 23 mos. Out of State: same
University of Colorado School of Medicine Denver, CO	In State: $8,200 for 36 mos. Out of State: $25,200 for 36 mos.
Quinnipiac College Hamden, CT	In State: $31,000 for 27 mos. Out of State: same
Yale University School of Medicine New Haven, CT	In State: $30,700 for 25 mos. Out of State: same
George Washington University Washington, DC	In State: N/A Out of State : $36,225 for 24 mos.
Howard University Washington, DC	In State: $19,250 for 24 mos. Out of State: same
Nova Southeastern University North Miami Beach, FL	In State: $13,500 per year Out of State: $15,500
University of Florida Gainesville, FL	In State: $4,035 for 22 mos. Out of State: $15,637 for 22 mos.
Emory University School of Medicine Atlanta, GA	In State: $26,500 for 28 mos. Out of State: same
Medical College of Georgia Augusta, GA	In State: $5,728 for 24 mos. Out of State: $16,752 for 24 mos.
Idaho State University Pocatello, ID	In State: $19,024 for 24 mos. Out of State: $34,768 for 24 mos.
Cook County Hospital/ Malcolm X College Chicago, IL	In State: $3,500 for 25 mos. Out of State: $10,600 for 25 mos.
Finch University of Health Sciences/The Chicago Medical School North Chicago, IL	In State: $30,000 for 24 mos. Out of State: same
Midwestern University Downers Grove, IL	In State: Bachelor's $8,528 per yr.; Master's $13,404 per yr.; Out of State: Bachelor's $11,544 per yr.; Master's $14,772 per yr.
Butler University/Methodist Hospital College of Pharmacy and Health Sciences Indianapolis, IN	In State: $33,700 for 21 mos. Out of State: same
Lutheran College of Health Professions Fort Wayne, IN	In State: $18,000 for 24 mos. Out of State: same

The University of Iowa College of Medicine Iowa City, IA	In State: $7,670 for 25 mos. Out of State: $23,965 for 25 mos.
University of Osteopathic Medicine & Health Sciences Des Moines, IA	In State: $18,900 for 24 mos. Out of State: same
Wichita State University College of Health Professions Wichita, KS	In State: $5,489 for 24 mos. Out of State: $16,993 for 24 mos.
University of Kentucky A.B. Chandler Medical Ctr. Lexington, KY	In State: $7,814 for 24 mos. Out of State: $19,715 for 24 mos.
Essex Community College Baltimore, MD	In County: $2,322 for 21 mos. In State: $3,954 for 21 mos. Out of State: $7,458 for 21 mos.
Northeastern University Boston, MA	In State: $19,200 for 24 mos. plus addl. fee for Master's option Out of State: same
University of Detroit Mercy Detroit, MI	In State: $28,350 for 24 mos. Out of State: same
Western Michigan University Kalamazoo, MI	In State: $10,419 for 24 mos. Out of State: $16,404 for 24 mos.
Augsburg College Minneapolis, MN	In State; $39,554 for 27 mos. Out of State: same
Saint Louis University School of Allied Health Professions St. Louis, MO	In State: $29,704 for 27 mos. Out of State: same
University of Nebraska Medical Center Omaha, NE	In State: $11,870 for 28 mos. Out of State: same
Rutgers University — University of Medicine and Dentistry of New Jersey Robert Wood Johnson Medical School Piscataway, NJ	In State: Master of Science: $222 per credit hour. Bachelor's: year 1, $3,786; year 2, $222 per credit hr. Out of State: Master's: $222 per hr. Bachelor's: year 1, $7,707; 2, $222 per credit hr.
Albany–Hudson Valley Albany Medical College Albany, NY	In State: $5,700 for 24 mos. Out of State: $11,600 for 24 mos.
Bayley Seton Hospital Staten Island, NY	In State: $17,600 for 23 mos. Out of State: same
Bronx Lebanon Hospital Center Bronx, NY	In State: $18,000 for 24 mos. Out of State: same
Brooklyn Hospital Center/Long Island University Brooklyn, NY	In State: $19,200 for 24 mos. Out of State: same

Catholic Medical Center
  Primary Care
Woodhaven, NY

In State: $24,500 for 23 mos.
Out of State: same

City University of New York
  Harlem Hospital Center
New York, NY

In State: $9,600 for 28 mos.
Out of State: $20,400 for 28 mos.

Cornell University Medical
  College
New York, NY

In State: $25,920 for 26 mos.
Out of State: same

D'Youville College
Buffalo, NY

In State: $9,420 per year
Out of State: same

Daemen College
Amherst, NY

In State: $10,000 for 48 mos.
Out of State: same

Rochester Institute of
  Technology
Rochester, NY

In State: $14,670 for 48 mos.
Out of State: same

State University of New York
  Health Science Center at
  Brooklyn
Brooklyn, NY

In State: $8,810 (commuter);
$11,215 (campus)
Out of State: $16,115 for 27 mos.

SUNY at Stony Brook
  School of Health Technology
  and Management
Stony Brook, NY

In State: $9,100 for 24 mos.
Out of State: $21,800 for 24 mos.

Touro College School of
  Health Sciences
Dix Hills, NY

In State: $22,400 for 24 mos.
Out of State: same

Bowman Gray School of
  Medicine of Wake Forest
  University
Winston-Salem, NC

In State: $24,000 for 24 mos.
Out of State: same

Duke University Medical
  Center
Durham, NC

In State: $33,600 for 25 mos.
Out of State: same

University of North Dakota
  School of Medicine
  Dept. of Community Medicine
  and Rural Health
Grand Forks, ND

In State: $7,000 for 12 mos.
Out of State: $8,000 for 12 mos.

Cuyahoga Community College
Parma, OH

In County: $6,200 for 22 mos.
In State: $7,500 for 22 mos.
Out of State: $12,800 for 22 mos.

Cuyahoga Community College
(major in surgery)
Parma, OH

In County: $6,370 for 22 mos.
In State; $7,700 for 22 mos.
Out of State: $13,100 for 22 mos.

Kettering College of Medical
  Arts
Kettering, OH

In State: $12,859 for 22 mos.
Out of State: same

University of Oklahoma
    Health Sciences Center
Oklahoma City, OK

In State: $11,000 for 30 mos.
Out of State: $32,000 for 30 mos.

Oregon Health Sciences
    University
Portland, OR

In State: $20,000 for 24 mos.
Out of State: $36,000 for 24 mos.

Duquesne University
    John G. Rangos, Sr., School
    of Health Sciences
Pittsburgh, PA

In State: $39,840 for 27 mos.
Out of state: same

Gannon University
Erie, PA

In State: $40,000 for 41 mos.
Out of State: same

King's College
Wilkes-Barre, PA

In State: $28,400 for 24 mos.
    (professional phase);
    $23,420 for pre-prof.
    phase for Bachelors
Out of State: same

Medical College of
    Pennsylvania and
    Hahnemann University
    School of Health Sciences &
    Humanities
Philadelphia, PA

In State: $25,000 for 24 mos.
Out of State: same

Philadelphia College of
    Textiles and Science
Philadelphia, PA

In State: $31,150 for 24 mos.
$55,630 for 44 mos.
Out of State: same

Saint Francis College
Loretto, PA

In State: $18,600 per year
Out of State: same

University of South Dakota
    School of Medicine
Vermillion, SD

In State: $11,700 for 24 mos.
Out of State: $19,700 for 24 mos.

Trevecca Nazarene University
Nashville, TN

In State: $28,017 for 24 mos.
Out of State: same

Baylor College of Medicine
Houston, TX

In State: $8,200 per yr.
Out of State: same

The University of Texas
    Medical Branch
    School of Allied Health
    Sciences
Galveston, TX

In State: $3,000 for 26 mos.
Out of State: $22,000 for 26 mos.

University of Texas
    Southwestern Medical
    Center at Dallas
Dallas, TX

In State: $3,450 for 27 mos.
Out of State: $20,585 for 27 mos.

University of Utah School of
    Medicine
Salt Lake City, UT

In State: $2,466.50 per qtr.
    (7 qtrs.)
Out of State: $2,874.00 per qtr.
    (7 qtrs.)

MEDEX Northwest University of Washington Seattle, WA	In State: $20,000 for 7 qtrs. Out of State: same
University of Wisconsin— Madison Madison, WI	In State: $2,549 per semester Out of State: $9,304 per semester MN Compact: $1,774.75 per se- mester

THE PLAN OF ACTION

I can still remember the butterflies that I felt in my stomach when I sent in my deposit to Yale. Reality set in: I'm going to PA school. Immediately, the thoughts raced in my head: I'm giving up my annual salary, plus I'm paying close to $14,000 a year for tuition, plus I'm borrowing money for living expenses, and to support my family. I began doing the math, and doubts crept in. But then, I remembered my goals, my focus, my plan.

I knew somehow things would work out. They did, and I don't regret one minute of it. In fact, I'm happier than I ever thought I'd be. I also fully recovered from the financial strain.

Here's how:

BUDGET

BE BRUTALLY HONEST WHEN MAKING YOUR BUDGET.

We've all heard this word before, and probably tried to write down our "income" on one side of a piece of paper and our "expenses" on the other. The problem is we usually have a lot more expenses than we're willing to write down; it's called denial. The only effective way to properly attempt a budget is to write down every penny you spend for an entire month. Everything counts, from dinner to clothes to a can of coke. If you're married, your spouse will have to participate, too. After 30 days, count up how much you actually spend and compare it to your original calculations. I think you'll be shocked at how much more you actually spend. But don't worry; now you can realistically see where all of your money is going and figure out ways to cut the fat.

To prepare you for some of the expenses you'll encounter when attending PA school, I've included a list of items that you'll most likely have to spend your money on:

- ▶ Rent/Mortgage
- ▶ Groceries
- ▶ Utilities
- ▶ Telephone
- ▶ Clothes
- ▶ Laundry/Dry Cleaning
- ▶ Entertainment
- ▶ Personal Expenses
- ▶ Transportation
- ▶ Parking
- ▶ Books
- ▶ Travel
- ▶ Insurance
- ▶ Medical Expenses
- ▶ Medical Equipment (stethoscope, otoscope)
- ▶ Child Care
- ▶ Credit Cards
- ▶ Miscellaneous
- ▶ Tuition
- ▶ Fees
- ▶ Other

EXPLORE YOUR OPTIONS

The biggest mistake I made in PA school, now that I look back, was quitting my part-time job at the hospital. Every program will tell you that you should not work while in school. You get so worked up about finally getting in that you want to do your best. You think that by not working you will be able to concentrate more on school. The problem is that if you're flat broke at the end of the semester, and your next check is weeks away, you can't concentrate anyway, so you might as well work. I gave up a part-time job which paid about $300 per week. Do some quick math and you'll see that's over $15,000 per year. Ouch! It still hurts to think about it.

But, on the other hand, if you really don't need the money, then definitely don't work. It will be especially hard to keep a job once you start clinical rotations. This is definitely a personal choice. All I'm trying to tell you is, use your own judgment; every program will tell you it's a bad idea, and that's not always true.

One last tip I'd like to share with you on this subject is that **everything is negotiable.** Six months before I graduated from school, I signed up for a job at a local hospital, received a $3,000 sign-on bonus (the next week), and got a check for $14,000 sent to the Yale Student Loan Department (tax free) for loan forgiveness. That's right, I negotiated a $17,000 bonus six months before I graduated. That $14,000 paid my last year's tuition, and the $3,000 sign-on bonus helped me and our family survive through graduation. Now, just as a side note, and to torture myself a little more, if I had kept my part-time job, too, that's $47,000 total.

How did I do that, you ask? Luck? Maybe. If you believe, like I do, that luck is when opportunity meets preparedness. The opportunities for PAs abound right now. "Six jobs for every graduate. . . ," "quit your job in the morning and have a new job by the afternoon." Our hospital is very PA friendly and always looking for PAs. They were planning on developing the cardiothoracic service and needed several PAs to fill slots (the opportunity was there). I interviewed with personnel and my current boss. I was then offered the position for the standard starting salary for all new grads, plus $7,000 in loan forgiveness, plus a $3,000 sign on bonus when I started work. Now, I wasn't too happy with the starting salary, and I was a little nervous about signing up for a job so early. In addition, I needed that sign-on bonus right now.

The next week I was back in the personnel office and I was told that the salary was firm. However, I got a little creative, and with my heart pounding and my stomach in my throat, I said, "I'm prepared to accept the job right now if you'll give me the sign-on bonus now, and double the loan forgiveness money." They accepted, and the rest is history. You see, the salary wasn't negotiable, but everything else was. Be creative, ask for the world—you deserve it. And most of all, don't forget to ask for loan forgiveness. Most employers will be happy to give it to you if you present it the right way.

By the way, one year after being with the hospital, the CT service was acquired by a private group, we received a significant raise, and everyone who joins the group gets loan forgiveness.

NEED-BASED AID

(Most of the following information pertains to graduate-level programs.)

You will hear the term "need-based aid" a lot once you begin filling out the vast number of financial aid forms. Need-based aid is available to

TO WORK, OR NOT TO WORK, THAT IS THE QUESTION.

help you finance your PA education. Since you and your family are expected to contribute to the cost of this education, this aid is supplementary.

Need Formula
Cost of Attendance − Student Contribution = Student Financial Need

As I mentioned above, once I got accepted to Yale, they assured me that I would have every opportunity to complete the program, regardless of ability to pay. This, in fact, is the underlying philosophy of need-based aid:

- ▶ Access: To a program that best suits your needs.
- ▶ Persistence: Inability to pay should not prevent you from finishing school.
- ▶ Fairness: Your family contribution will be determined fairly.

WHO IS AN INDEPENDENT STUDENT?

Until July 23, 1992, all graduate students were considered independent, for federal aid purposes, if you were over 24 years old, or were under 24 and not claimed as a dependent on anyone's income tax statement for the first calendar year in which you were seeking aid.

However, most schools will ask for parental information even if you are totally independent and left the nest 20 years ago. You will be asked to obtain from your parents tax returns, CD information, bank account numbers, etc.

I personally did not ask my mom for any information. But, since I did not submit any of her financial records, I left myself at risk for not receiving certain funds. In other words, if there was money left over after all the other students with need who did submit parental information, then I could receive that same aid. By the way, there was money left over and I received all that I needed.

HOW IS NEED DETERMINED?

Most PA programs should provide you with a budget worksheet which you can use to determine your cost of attendance for that institution. Below is a sample worksheet.

BUDGET WORKSHEET

INCOME	CURRENT MONTHLY	PROJECTED MONTHLY
Student/Spouse Income		
Student/Spouse Resources		
Parental Support		
Financial Aid	_____	_____
EDUCATION EXPENSES		
Tuition		
Mandatory Fees		
Books, Magazines, and Papers		
Equipment	_____	_____

	CURRENT MONTHLY	PROJECTED MONTHLY

HOUSING AND HOUSING MAINTENANCE

Rent/Mortgages

Utilities

Gas/Oil

Electric

Water

Telephone _____ _____

FOOD AND GROCERIES

Food

Groceries/Household Items

Snacks, "Coffee" Breaks, Lunch _____ _____

TRANSPORTATION

Gasoline

Car Maintenance

Bus Fares

Insurance _____ _____

PERSONAL

Clothing

Grooming (Haircuts, etc.)

Dry Cleaning

Laundry

Other _____ _____

MEDICAL

Insurance

Doctors

Dentists

Medication

Other _____ _____

ENTERTAINMENT

Meals Away from Home

Movies/Concerts

Other _____ _____

CHILD CARE

Day Care/Nursery School

Babysitter

Child Support _____ _____

TOTAL EXPENSES _____ _____

FUNDS AVAILABLE/ SURPLUS _____ _____

NEED ANALYSIS

Your financial contribution is based on a congressional formula called Congressional Methodology (CM). Need analysis is a process used to estimate how much you will need to supplement your theoretically available resources. The two components include cost of attendance and an estimate of your family's ability to contribute.

CONGRESSIONAL METHODOLOGY (CM)

Uses taxable and nontaxable base-year income to calculate the expected student contribution (SC).

STUDENT CONTRIBUTION (SC)

This is the amount you and your spouse are expected to contribute to finance your education. This amount is the same for all schools. Once this figure is determined, it is subtracted from the cost of attendance, and the remaining amount is your financial need.

The resources used to calculate the SC include items like savings, school year earnings, and spousal income. Your expected contribution is based on an analysis of your income and asset information, size of household, and number of family members in college.

Students are expected to contribute 35% of their assets each year to meet educational needs.

PARENTAL CONTRIBUTION (PC)

Includes calculations based on parental income, expenses, and assets. Income includes items like social security, welfare, and dividends, as well as job salaries.

PROFESSIONAL JUDGMENT

About now you may be asking, "Does anyone, besides a computer, ever look at my financial information and make a personal decision based on my circumstances?" The answer is yes. The financial aid counselor knows that even though you made $30,000 last year, you will lose some, or all, of that income this year. They will use their professional judgment when allowing or disallowing certain funds. Needless to say, make friends with someone in the financial aid office quickly.

ORGANIZE YOUR FINANCIAL RECORDS

SUGGESTIONS

1. Follow instructions on every form.
2. Copy all forms.
3. Keep folders on each school.
4. Keep copies of last two years' taxes.
5. Gather all account numbers on bank statements, stocks, mutual funds, etc.
6. Obtain all signatures from parents, spouse, etc.
7. Put name and social security number on all pages.
8. Respond immediately to all requests from lenders.
9. Follow up on everything.
10. Report any change in status immediately.

FEDERAL FINANCIAL AID (TITLE IV & TITLE IX)

TITLE IV

Part of the Higher Education Act, to qualify for this federal money you must meet the following requirements:

1. Be enrolled as a student in a specific program.
2. Be a U.S. citizen or eligible non-citizen.
3. Be making satisfactory progress in your course of study.
4. Neither be in default nor owe a refund for any federal aid received in the past.
5. Be enrolled at least half-time (6 semester hours).

Address questions to:

▶ Federal Student Aid Information Center Hotline
1-800-333-INFO
▶ 301-369-0518 (a TDD number for hearing impaired)

Use this number to check and explain schools which participate, eligibility requirements, how awards are determined, complaints, the verification process, and to order publications.

TITLE IX

The purpose of these programs is to encourage and support graduate and professional programs to provide incentives and support for U.S. citizens, especially women and under-represented groups, to complete Master's and doctoral programs. These programs are divided into six parts, A–G, although only parts A–C apply to PA programs.

Part A

Grants to Institutions and Consortia to Encourage Women and Minority Participation in Graduate Education
These grants are made to schools to help them identify talented **undergraduates** who demonstrate financial need.

Part B

Patricia Roberts Harris Fellowships Program
Provided to the schools to distribute among master's, doctoral, and professional students. Distributed as follows to **minority students and women:**

▶ 50% Master's and professional study
▶ 50% fellowship for doctoral study

Part C

Jacob Javits Fellowship
Available for graduate students studying in the arts, humanities, and social science.

▶ **Contact:** Ms. Diana Haymond, Director
Jacob Javits Fellowship Program
U.S. Department of Education
400 Maryland Avenue, SW, ROB-3
Washington, DC 20202-5251
(202) 708-9415

Note: The preceding programs may or may not be available to you as a PA student. Please check with your individual schools about your eligibility.

OTHER FEDERAL GRANT PROGRAMS*

Department of Health and Human Services (HHS), National Institutes of Health (NIH)—Public Health Service Commission Corps (COSTEP)

This is a service-related award. You will be assigned to one of eight Public Health Agencies, and be required to provide clinical or research services, for a monthly stipend of $1,950 for a single person. Deadlines for the COSTEP applications are December 31, for positions May 1 through August 31, May 1 for positions September 1 through December 31, and October 1 for positions January 1 through April 30. You will be eligible to participate in this program during your clinical phase.

▶ Contact: COSTEP
PHS Recruitment
8201 Greensboro Drive
Suite 600
McLean, VA 22102
(800) 221-9393

NATIONAL HEALTH SERVICE CORPS (NHSC)

An excellent program, this award covers tuition and provides you with a monthly stipend. You will incur a two-year obligation to a designated area (under-served). You will be given several sites to select from throughout the country. You will be required to make contact with these sites for availability and to negotiate a salary. Four hundred awards are given out per year. You must fill out a questionnaire and application to be considered for an award. I personally applied, but was rejected. However, I know several people who received awards.

▶ Contact: NHSC Scholarships
8201 Greensboro Drive, #600
McLean, VA 22102
(800) 221-9393
In VA: (703) 734-6855

INDIAN HEALTH SERVICE (IHS)

A minimum two-year obligation for two years of financial support. Priority is given to Indian students, but others may apply.

▶ Contact: IHS Scholarship office at: (800) 962-2817

DEPARTMENT OF VETERANS AFFAIRS HEALTH PROFESSIONAL SCHOLARSHIP PROGRAM

▶ Contact: (202) 565-7528 for more information

FEDERAL LOAN PROGRAMS

FEDERAL STAFFORD STUDENT LOAN PROGRAM (FORMERLY GSL)

These loans are offered through your bank, credit union, or other lending institutions. Graduate students may borrow up to $8,500 per year up to a

* First come, first served, so apply early.

total of $65,500. To qualify for a Stafford loan, you must demonstrate financial need as determined by the CM formula mentioned above.

The interest rate is 8% for new borrowers, after July 1, 1987, and goes up to 10% after the fifth year of repayment. These loans are based on need, not creditworthiness; therefore, no co-signer is necessary.

Sample Repayment Table for Stafford loan:

If your interest rate is 8%: # months to pay in full

Loan Amount	60	72	84	96	108	120
$1,000	20.28	17.54	15.59	14.14	13.02	12.14
5,000	101.39	87.67	77.94	70.69	65.10	60.67
6,000	121.66	105.20	93.52	84.83	78.12	72.80
6,500	131.80	113.97	101.32	91.90	84.63	78.87
7,500	152.08	131.50	116.90	106.03	97.65	91.00

FEDERAL PERKINS LOAN (FORMERLY NATIONAL DIRECT STUDENT LOAN)

This is a good loan, currently at 5% interest, available to undergraduate and graduate students. You apply for this loan, and you get the money from your individual school rather than the bank. You can borrow up to $5,000 per year for a maximum of $30,000. To qualify for this loan, you must demonstrate financial need as determined by your financial aid application. This is the loan that you may not receive if you fail to include your parents' information on your application.

Sample Repayment for Federal Perkins Loan

Total Indebtedness	Number of Payments	Monthly Payment	Total interest Charges	Total Repaid
$4,500	120	$ 47.73	$1,227.60	$5,727.60
9,000	120	95.46	2,455.20	11,455.20
18,000	120	190.92	4,910.40	22,910.40

Source: US Department of Education

FEDERAL SUPPLEMENTAL LOAN FOR STUDENTS (SLS)

These loans are not as desirable as the above two programs; however, they can be a great source of money if you need more than you can get with the above programs. You obtain these loans from a commercial lender, with the interest rate being tied to the 52-week treasury bill (T-Bill) not to exceed 11%. You may borrow up to $ 10,000 per year to a maximum of $73,000. The loan amount is based on your educational costs minus any other financial aid you receive.

STATE PROGRAMS

State programs include loan forgiveness, for which you work at a designated clinic or site in an under-served area, and receive up to $20,000 in loan forgiveness. Another program is the Health Profession Shortage Area (HPSA), which provides loans at a dollar-for-dollar match for educational loans.

▶ Contact: NHSC
Site Development and Placement Branch
4350 East-West Highway, 8th floor
Bethesda, MD 20814
(301) 594-4165
Fax: (301) 594-4077

CONSTITUENT CHAPTERS

Most of the state chapters of the AAPA offer some sort of scholarship program for students. Contact your local program to see if they have anything available. Join the state organization while you're at it.

OTHER

For a Physician Assistant Student Financial Aid Information Booklet, sponsored by the AAPA, write to:

▶ SpecWorks
810 S. Bond St.
Baltimore, MD 21231
1-800-708-7581 (8:30 am–6:00 pm EST)
Fax: 410/558-1410 (24 hours)

Ask for publication #124

GOOD LUCK IN YOUR SEARCH FOR FINANCIAL AID.

PA Job Descriptions

This chapter is designed to introduce the PA school applicant to the various clinical specialties and disciplines in which PAs practice. We will cover the seven areas of clinical medicine (Family Practice, Emergency Medicine, Pediatrics, Psychiatry, OB-GYN, Internal Medicine, and Surgery) which many programs require as mandatory rotations.

Each of the above specialties will be described as follows:

1. *Description of Duties*
2. *The Team*
3. *Salary*
4. *Summary*

The *Description of Duties* is an account of the day-to-day activities and functions of a PA working in a given specialty. We will point out the various clinical presentations and types of patients you can expect to evaluate and treat in that particular discipline, and try to give you a sense of the physical and mental challenges associated with the job. For instance, some areas of medicine are more cerebral than others, while other specialties tend to be more task and procedure oriented.

After reading over the various job descriptions, the reader may come to some insightful conclusions. For instance, you may be surprised to find out that the traditional Family Practice PA doesn't necessarily get to spend a great deal of time with his or her patients, as reported in most of the PA literature. Many Family Practice PAs are so busy that they barely have time for lunch. You may be surprised to find out that the Surgery PA actually has more of an opportunity to get to know the patient, and the patient's family, much better since he or she may have that patient on his/her service for several days.

I bring up the above point because the premise of this book is to set yourself apart from the competition. Many applicants come to the interview without a clue as to how real PAs function. They think we have unlimited time to spend with our patients. It's very refreshing, and it shows a great deal of insight, when an applicant is knowledgeable about the different jobs we perform and knows that what the literature says and what we actually do may be two different things.

During the course of interviews, 90% of applicants will tell you that they want to work in "Family Practice" or "with AIDS patients." They think that this is the politically correct answer. They fail to realize, however, that the people interviewing them are real PAs working in a variety of specialties. Less than 40% of all PAs work in Family Practice; that leaves 60% of all PAs to work in other areas. We need PAs in every specialty. I can't tell you how many applicants will come to the interview with, for example, six years of orthopedic experience and then tell you that they want to work in an AIDS clinic. That may be a legitimate goal for some, but most are not being true to the committee, or themselves. The key is to be consistent and to be honest. Don't fake it, because it won't work!

The Team consists of the professionals you will interact with the most on a daily basis. Our profession is one in which we must work in collaboration with a variety of medical, and non-medical, personnel. The closer you keep the "team concept" to your understanding of our profession, the better off you'll be at interview time.

The ***Salary*** is self-explanatory. We simply try to give you an idea of the earning potential of PAs in a variety of settings. Of course, these numbers will vary depending on the type of practice (hospital versus clinic versus private practice) and your negotiating skills.

The ***Summary*** is a quick and concise synopsis of the stress level, hours, educational opportunities, research opportunities, and pace of the job. The summary also gives you an overall "gestalt" for which type of person generally gravitates towards each specialty.

FAMILY PRACTICE

Description of Duties. This area is the cornerstone of our profession; approximately 40% of all PAs work in Family Practice. The Family Practice PA may work in a clinic (urban or rural) or for a private physician or group of physicians. PAs working in Family Practice generally require a strong breadth of knowledge in the following areas: Pediatrics, Internal Medicine, Dermatology, Orthopedics, HIV, Cardiology, Endocrinology, Pulmonology, OB-GYN, and Renal Disease. In addition, he/she must develop the skills to perform minor surgery, splint and cast limbs, and remove foreign bodies from eyes, to name just a few.

The patients seen in a Family Practice setting are generally non-acute, except, perhaps, in a rural setting where you may be the only provider for miles. Many of the patients are known to the clinic or practice and present with colds, flu, and minor ailments. Others, however, may be more complex and require closer follow-up. Depending on the type and location of the practice, you may follow a great number of HIV and AIDS patients. You may also be required to go out into the community and provide care to the indigent population. In fact, many inner city clinics cater specifically to this population.

In addition to the various acute illnesses evaluated and treated on a daily basis, there is also a very routine part to this job. For instance, the PA performs numerous school, sports, and well-baby physical examinations. Many patients are diabetic or hypertensive and require periodic, routine follow-up visits. Giving immunizations and vaccines is also an important part of this job.

Of course, like all specialties, the Family Practice PA works very closely with his/her supervising physician(s). Although the PA works fairly autonomously in this setting, the physician is always available for consultation on the more difficult cases.

Most Family Practice clinics have a pharmacy and/or lab on-site. Some will also have x-ray capabilities. Depending on the size and budget of the facility, the PA may be required to perform basic laboratory studies to confirm or rule out a diagnosis.

Contrary to popular belief (of many PA school applicants), a PA working in a Family Practice setting doesn't always have vast amounts of time to spend with his or her patients. In fact, many PAs in a busy practice will see over 40 patients per day, often skipping lunch to stay on schedule. Generally, however, the hours are nine to five, and there typically is no call or weekend duty.

The Team. The Family Practice team varies from office to office depending on the size of the practice. In general, PAs work alongside of physicians, nurse practitioners, nurses, medical assistants, and clerical personnel. A larger practice may also employ x-ray technicians, laboratory technicians, and pharmacists.

Salary. Depending on the type of practice (solo versus group versus clinic), Family Practice PAs probably average in the middle of the salary range; from $50,000 to $75,000 per year. Of course, salary is dependent on the amount of clinical experience the clinician has. Some clinics are open during the evening hours and on weekends, which may provide an opportunity for moonlighting and earning extra income. This could add another $3,000 to $10,000 to the total income.

Summary. Family Practice represents a traditional role for PAs. This setting provides a great opportunity for the PA to enhance his/her clinical skills by evaluating and treating a variety of medical presentations. Although the job is not as leisurely paced as one may expect, the stress level is usually very manageable as the patients tend to be non-acute. The job has the potential to become routine at times, but certainly not boring.

EMERGENCY MEDICINE

Description of Duties. About 8% of Physician Assistants work in this exciting arena. Generally, an Emergency Room (ER) is divided into several sections: surgery, medicine, trauma, major medical, fast track, pediatrics, and psychiatry. Some PAs will work in primarily one area, but many rotate through them all depending on preference, experience, and hospital policy.

In the surgery section, the patients usually have obvious complaints and injuries, and the PA's role is highly procedure oriented; he/she does a lot of suturing, splinting/casting, removing foreign bodies from eyes, and wrapping sprains and strains. However, some patients may have more insidious complaints, which involve further diagnostic work-up with x-rays and laboratory testing; such as appendicitis, bowel obstructions, and kidney/gallstones.

In the medicine section, the PA sees a variety of common and complex patients with complaints of asthma, fever, shortness of breath, nausea/vomiting, dizziness, etc. Many of the patients are elderly and have a history of diabetes or heart disease. The PA usually works very closely with the patient's family physician, especially when the patient has a complicated past medical history. This area of the ER is less task/procedure oriented, and the PA is challenged to collect a thorough medical history and utilize excellent clinical skills to arrive at a diagnosis.

The trauma section of the ER is reserved for acute injuries sustained from motor vehicle accidents, gunshot wounds, falls, knife wounds, fights, ruptured aneurysms, and burns, to name a few. In this arena the PA will have a specific task as a member of the trauma team. Usually, a surgeon will head the team, and the PA will perform duties such as collecting blood gases, putting in a chest tube, holding pressure on an arterial bleeder, or helping insert a central line. Not all PAs who work in the ER are directly involved with the trauma team. In fact, many hospitals require additional training for the PA who wants to work in this area.

Major medicine is an area in which patients in need of acute medical attention are treated. Usually, heart attack victims and patients in acute respiratory distress, or cardiac arrest, are triaged to this area. The PA may be the initial provider on the scene and will be responsible to initiate treatment until the attending physician arrives.

Fast track is an area designated for follow up visits and routine, minor illnesses like sore throats, coughs, hangnails, etc. This is usually staffed by a designated PA on a daily basis, or by several PAs who rotate through on different days.

The pediatric section of the ER is usually covered by the pediatric residents, interns, or PAs. The patient's ages range from newborn babies to teenagers. Common presentations include asthma attacks, sore throats, ear infections, and fevers. Obviously, the clinicians work closely with the patient's pediatrician when forming a treatment plan. Usually, the surgical residents will handle the lacerations and broken bones.

Most ERs also have a psychiatric room/section for patients with acute psychiatric problems. In addition, the same area is generally used for intoxicated patients or highly uncooperative/combative patients. The PA has a limited role in this area, except to contact psychiatry and have the patient evaluated. The PA may have to treat lacerations, bruises, or acute overdoses prior to the psychiatric evaluation.

The Team. The team in the ER consists of a variety of clinicians, technicians, nurses, clerical personnel, security, and personnel from various emergency medical services. PAs work very closely with the attending physicians, housestaff, consulting physicians, nurses, and technicians to ensure the best treatment for the patient.

Salary. ER PAs tend to be at the higher end of the pay scale, in part due to the stress of the job, but also due to the number of hours and various shifts worked. The range is from $50,000 to $80,000 per year.

Summary. The ER PA must be able to work in a stressful environment in collaboration with a variety of team members. The job is fast-paced, and calls for a clinician who has both excellent surgical skills and a thorough medical knowledge. Although there is usually a lot of back-up available, due to the usually high patient volume, many ER PAs work autonomously, requiring little supervision.

PEDIATRICS

Description of Duties. Pediatric PAs comprise about 3% of the PA population, and either work in clinics, private pediatrician offices, or in a hospital setting. In this section we will cover the Pediatric/Neonatal Physician Assistant in the hospital setting, i.e., the housestaff.

The Pediatric/Neonatal PA functioning as Housestaff implies, by its very name, duties divided into and covering several areas and specialties. You are required to see patients on the in-patient pediatric floor, attend and assist with high-risk deliveries, evaluate and manage newborns (from 30 weeks' gestation on up), work in the pediatric clinic, and provide coverage to the emergency room as needed.

Usually, the job requires in-house calls and rotating shifts, as well as night and weekend coverage. As housestaff, you may be the only clinician available for emergencies during the middle of the night. Although the attending physician is always available by phone, you will often be the first clinician on the scene to evaluate and stabilize the patient.

In pediatrics, the patients are usually admitted through the emergency room or directly from a pediatrician's office. Your duties upon admission include performing a history and physical examination, ordering necessary tests, forming a diagnosis and treatment plan, and consulting with the attending pediatrician. You may also be required to draw blood samples, catheterize patients, and perform lumbar punctures. You then follow the patient on a daily basis, writing progress notes and discussing further diagnostic and treatment modalities with the attending pediatrician.

In Neonatology, the PA medically manages newborns from 30 weeks gestation until term. The supervising physician in this area is a neonatologist. Again, as housestaff, your responsibility is to manage the day-to-day medical care of these neonates who have a variety of acute and chronic problems. This service is very procedure oriented, with plenty of intravenous starts, lumbar punctures, central (intravenous) line placements, ventilator management, collecting blood gases, placing chest tubes, and much more.

Attending high-risk deliveries is also a part of Neonatology. Here, you are responsible for resuscitation of the newborn in the delivery room. Many times you are working autonomously, with only you and the nursing staff responsible to revive the infant until the anesthesiologist and pediatrician arrive.

The pediatric clinic is usually reserved for scheduled, non-emergent patients. This is where the PA performs well baby check-ups, gives immunizations, and sees a variety of colds, earaches, and sore throats. The acuity of the patients is not as high as in neonatology, but the pace can be fast and furious.

Common calls to the emergency room are for asthma attacks, broken bones, and high fevers. On occasion, however, you may see a patient suffering from cardiac arrest or an acute overdose. In addition, many families without medical insurance will bring their children to the emergency room for routine visits: colds, coughs, and rashes. Surgical injuries are usually deferred to the surgical PAs or housestaff.

The Team. The pediatric team consists of pediatricians, neonatologists, residents, interns, physician assistants, nurses, respiratory therapists, occupational therapists, nurse's aides, unit clerks, and secretaries.

Salary. Pediatric PAs tend to be at the lower end of the pay scale with respect to PAs in other specialties. The range is from $50,000 to $75,000 depending on the hours worked.

Summary. This is a job in which there is a lot of calm, followed by moments of chaos. You must be willing, and able, to work various shifts, including nights, weekends, and holidays. The stress level ranges from extremely high when dealing with critically ill newborns to fairly routine when working in the clinic. You need to be well organized, and, at times, ready to be in two places at one time. This is not a job for the PA lacking in confidence and maturity.

PSYCHIATRY

Description of Duties. Psychiatry PAs generally work in either a hospital-based setting or in a clinic/mental health center. Approximately 3% of all PAs work in psychiatry.

In the hospital setting, PAs will either work on a consultation service or on the psychiatric ward of the facility. On the consultation (consult) service, the PA will be called to evaluate in-patients from any area of the hospital—surgery or medicine. Working closely with the psychiatrist in this setting, the PA will evaluate patients for depression, anxiety, alcohol withdrawal, psychiatric medication problems, dementia, delirium, and, quite common to elderly Intensive Care Unit patients, "sun-downing." Many of these patients have a history of psychiatric illness and simply need to be followed while in the hospital. Others, however, may present with new symptoms and may require a more detailed work-up.

Once the patient is seen and evaluated, the PA discusses the case with his/her attending or hospital-based psychiatrist and consults with the patient's attending physician as to the recommendation. Many times the recommendation is to change a medication or simply hold it for a period of time. Occasionally, the PA will recommend further testing, especially with patients who present with new findings. The PA may recommend a neurology consult or an MRI or CT scan to rule out certain pathology.

The PA will then follow all of the patients on the consult service, usually daily, writing notes and continuing recommendations until the patient is discharged or stable enough to not warrant further consultation.

PAs working in the psychiatric ward of the hospital and a clinic/mental health center have similar duties and will be covered together here. Many of these clinics treat a great deal of substance abuse patients (alcohol and drug) and patients considered to have "dual diagnosis" (substance abuse and psychiatric illness), for example, a patient suffering from alcoholism and schizophrenia. The patients may be treated on an in-patient or out-patient basis. The PA's role in this area is usually to take care of the patient's medical needs: physical exams, monitor the patient's non-psychiatric medications, hypertension, diabetes, seizures, etc. The PA may also be responsible to give classes to the patients on topics such as AIDS, hepatitis, and nutrition.

Some PAs work in this area because of the opportunity to be involved in research. Many clinics offer experimental drugs and/or treatment programs to the patients who are struggling with alcohol or drug problems, and who have failed conventional treatment. The PA is more involved with the patient's psychiatric disease in this setting, and may be more involved in counseling and group therapy than the medical aspect of the treatment plan.

The Team. In a hospital setting (consult service), the PA works closely with the hospital psychiatrists, the patient's family, the nursing staff, and the patient's attending physician. In the clinic setting, the team consists of psychiatrists, psychologists, social workers, counselors, nurses, attending physicians (occasionally), technicians, and clerical personnel.

The Salary. Psychiatry PAs tend to be at the low range of the pay scale. The salary range is from $50,000 to $65,000.

Summary. This position is generally one of low stress. The hospital-based consult service PA works fairly autonomously, depending on his/her supervisor, and sees a variety of patients throughout the hospital. The PA working in the psychiatric clinic usually works at a slow pace and can have a tedious job at times. This may be the perfect opportunity, however, for the PA interested in doing research and publishing papers.

OB-GYN

Description of Duties. The OB-GYN specialty is traditionally filled by female PAs and represents about 3% of the PA workforce. This specialty deals with both obstetrics (dealing with pregnant women during pregnancy and childbirth) and gynecology (dealing with diseases peculiar to women, primarily those of the genital tract as well as endocrinology and reproductive physiology). In this section we will discuss the role of the hospital-based OB-GYN PA.

This position is one of great diversity with respect to the various practice settings. The OB-GYN PA may work in the hospital OB-GYN clinic, the operating room, the in-patient OB-GYN floor, the maternity ward, and, where applicable, in a community van which reaches out to the indigent population in the community.

In the OB-GYN clinic, the PA will see women for prenatal visits, annual Pap smears, pregnancy testing, and a variety of complaints relative to the female anatomy. The PA should be proficient in the pelvic examination. The OB-GYN PA should also have excellent communication skills, as many of the patients are teenagers and require a great deal of counseling with respect to teen pregnancy, HIV prevention, and sexually transmitted disease prevention.

In the operating room, the PA is usually a first or second assistant to the attending OB-GYN physician. The majority of surgical cases include hysterectomies and laparoscopic explorations of the pelvic cavity. PAs may also have a role in assisting the attending physician in cesarean section deliveries.

The in-patient OB-GYN floor is generally reserved for patients recovering from surgery. The PA's role is to round on all of the patients, change dressings, check labs, write progress notes, and write orders. This function is very similar to that of the surgical PA.

The maternity ward is, of course, where most of the deliveries take place. PAs generally have a limited role on this floor. Most babies are delivered by the attending physician, or by midwifes who play a significant role in many hospitals.

Some hospitals, or clinics, will have a community van which goes out into various neighborhoods and provides routine and prenatal care to mothers who would not ordinarily come to a facility. This may be the only medical care many of these patients ever receive. This is an excellent opportunity for the PA to reach out and make a difference in the community.

The Team. For obvious reasons, the OB-GYN field is predominantly comprised of females, except for attending physicians. In addition to PAs and

MDs, the team may consist of nurse practitioners, nurse midwifes, nurses, technicians, OR personnel, and clerical personnel.

Salary: OB-GYN PAs tend to earn average salaries with respect to PAs in other areas. The range is from $50,000 to $70,000.

Summary. This specialty is traditionally filled by female PAs. There is a great amount of diversity in OB-GYN, ie, surgery, medicine, in-patient, and clinic responsibilities. This job can be both physically and mentally challenging, requiring both excellent diagnostic skills and proficient surgical capabilities.

SURGERY

Description of Duties. Surgery and its related subspecialties comprise an area second only to internal medicine in terms of total numbers of PA positions (approximately 22%). Physician assistants function effectively in multiple clinical settings, performing in-hospital surgical tasks along with and, not infrequently, in place of residents. Many hospitals employ PAs as house officers (housestaff) in lieu of maintaining a surgical residency teaching program comprised of MDs.

Physician assistants who wish to pursue a career in surgery should be proficient in medicine. The answer to this apparent paradox becomes clear with an examination of PA responsibilties on a typical hospital surgical service. PAs, as house officers, are responsible for the preoperative, intraoperative, and postoperative care of surgical patients. A given patient's preoperative state of health clearly will affect his/her intraoperative and postoperative care, as well as the overall prognosis. Timely identification of any pre-existing conditions (diabetes mellitus, pulmonary disease, coronary artery disease, peripheral vascular disease, renal disease, liver disease, or compromise in the immune system), together with appropriate preoperative intervention, are critical to a favorable outcome. Similarly, there are a myriad of postoperative conditions which can arise: fever, pulmonary embolus, respiratory distress, renal failure, infection, and hemorrhage. These conditions can be lessened, or prevented, by the intervention of the knowledgeable surgical PA.

The responsibilities of the surgical PA include taking the patient's history, performing the physical exam, ordering appropriate preoperative laboratory tests and x-rays, writing the admission orders, and performing a preoperative check prior to the patient's surgery. In addition, postoperatively, the PA rounds on the floor, writes notes on all of the patients, changes the treatment plan as needed, and consults with the attending physician (surgeon) on a daily basis.

Intraoperatively, the PA's duties include first and second assisting. Many surgical procedures consist of the attending surgeon and the PA to do the actual surgery, with the ancillary help of the scrub nurse, circulating nurse, technicians, and anesthesiologist. The surgical PA should have a thorough knowledge of anatomy and be technically proficient in various procedures.

In addition to assisting with major surgical procedures, the surgical PA should be able to perform a variety of minor surgical and invasive procedures. These include, but are not limited to, administering local anesthesia, surgical debridement of wounds, intramuscular injections and arthrocentesis, peripheral and central venous cannulation, chest tube placement/ removal, proper immobilization of various fractured bones (as well as traction where indicated), bladder catheterization and cystometrograms, and airway management/intubation. The surgical PA should also be able to perform and interpret electrocardiograms and be Adult Cardiac Life Support (ACLS) qualified.

The surgical PA is often called to the emergency room to evaluate and admit patients to the surgical service. The ability of the surgical PA to work in collaboration with the ER team is essential. Decisions made by the PA affect not only the patient's health, but also the efforts of the nurses, lab technicians, respiratory therapists, physical and occupational therapists, and team members from other services in the hospital.

The surgical PA is usually required to take call on a rotating basis. This usually involves spending the night in the hospital, mostly in the Surgical Intensive Care Unit, but providing care to the entire service as needed.

The Team. The surgical team consists of a variety of medical and surgical personnel. Mostly, the PA works with attending surgeons, nurses, various technicians and therapists, circulating nurses, scrub nurses, and anesthesiologists (or nurse anesthetists) in the operating room, along with medical attendings, and various interns and residents.

The Salary. Surgery PAs are usually on the higher end of the pay scale. This is usually due to the acuity of the patients, the hours on call, and the ability of the attending to be reimbursed for first assistant services. The range is from $50,000 to over $100,000.

Summary. This is definitely not the job for the shy and retiring. The surgical PA is generally a "Type A" individual. In addition, he or she must have excellent written and verbal communication skills, a willingness to handle responsibility, and the ability to be a team player. He or she must also be able to pay strict attention to detail.

INTERNAL MEDICINE

Description of Duties. Approximately 8% of practicing PAs work in internal medicine. In this section we will cover the hospital-based internal medicine PA. The reader should keep in mind, however, that there are many opportunities available for PAs to work with private physicians and group practices.

The medicine PA must have, or acquire, a general understanding of all the medical subspecialties: cardiology, renal medicine, pulmonology, endocrinology, neurology, dermatology, hematology, and HIV medicine. As a result, medicine makes a great first job for the new graduate who wants to build a solid foundation for future practice.

In the hospital environment, the medicine PA is usually a part of a team with other PAs and the housestaff (residents and interns). Quite commonly, a medical student or PA student will be assigned to the service also.

The typical day usually starts early in the morning with individual rounds. Each clinician will briefly see and examine his/her patients. Next comes team rounds. The chief resident will gather the team and discuss each patient on the service. This usually takes place just outside of each patient's room. If the patient is new to the service, admitted overnight, the primary provider will give a brief, but thorough, summary of the patient's history and physical examination, laboratory results, x-ray results, diagnosis, and treatment plan. The chief residents may then question the team, or an individual member, about issues relevant to the patient's case or presentation. This procedure is affectionately called "pimping," and it is a way to keep the entire team on its toes and makes for a great daily learning experience. Morning rounds can last from two to three hours depending on the size of the service and the mood of the chief resident.

After team rounds, the PA will generally have some time to check lab results and tests, and read notes in his/her patient's charts which may have been written by consultants or the patient's attending physician. The PA will then check any lab results or tests which may have been pending and begin to write the daily note on each patient. Included in the notes is the plan for the day and any specific orders that must be carried out as part of that treatment plan.

Throughout the day, the PA touches base with attending physicians and consulting physicians with respect to the patient's progress and treatment plan. The PA will also discuss any significant findings with the chief resident, as he/she is ultimately responsible for the service.

At some point in the day, the team will meet again for x-ray rounds. An attending radiologist usually presides over the meeting, in the Department of Radiology, and will discuss each and every x-ray, ultrasound, MRI, angiogram, or CT scan which was performed on the patients on your service that morning. This is a great learning experience and helps the clinician get better acquainted with reading and interpreting various radiological studies.

In addition to team rounds and radiology rounds, the team may also have "attending rounds." Usually, one of the attending physicians is assigned to your service for the month, and may give two or three lectures a week on various medical topics. This may include visiting with some patients and discussing his/her clinical findings. Again, this is an excellent and valuable learning tool.

Each clinician is usually assigned one or two new admissions per day. The PA will go to the emergency room and perform a complete history and physical exam on the patient. He/she will then order any appropriate tests (labs, x-rays, etc.), touch base with the attending physician, and write the patient's admission orders. The patient is presented and discussed with the rest of the team at morning rounds.

In addition to the daily routine described above, the medicine PA must also be proficient in various diagnostic and therapeutic procedures; obtaining blood gases, performing lumbar punctures, starting IVs, drawing blood, central line placement, and thoracentesis. Usually, the chief resident will teach these various procedures to the PA and allow him/her to accomplish them as proficiency and comfort level progress.

The Team. The internal medicine team consists of PAs, residents, interns, nurses, attending physicians, consulting physicians, technicians, aides, and clerical personnel.

Salary. The salary for internal medicine PAs tends to be on the low side; this is usually due to the excellent hours and great teaching opportunities. The range is from $50,000 to $65,000.

Summary. This specialty offers great hours and low stress. In addition, this is a good job for the new graduate because of the excellent learning opportunities available. Many PAs will stay in this position for a couple of years and then move on to private practice, or specialize in one of the sub-specialties. This is definitely the perfect position for the cerebral-minded PA.

GRIEVING

For those of you who have taken classes in "Death and Dying," you will be familiar with the five steps involved in the grieving process: denial, anger, bargaining, depression, and acceptance. While being rejected from PA school does not compare with losing a family member, or perhaps even with losing a pet, it can still be a devastating and discouraging experience. The trick is to move through the process and get to the acceptance phase as quickly as possible. This will allow you to begin working toward improving your application for next year.

At first, you will have a hard time believing the fact that, after all of the hard work you put into the process, you weren't accepted. You may then become angry, realizing that your best-laid plans have been shattered. Your attitude may become self-defeating. The key here is not to burn any bridges, and by no means should you call the program and try to bargain, or beg, for acceptance. This will only hurt your chances for next year. Believe me, there will be a next year and it will come sooner than you think.

You will naturally be depressed, but you will eventually come to accept the fact that you didn't get in and that the sun will still rise tomorrow. Don't take things too personally, as many excellent candidates don't get into PA school on their first try. It's mostly a matter of logistics: too many good applicants for precious few slots. Work through the process and get ready to go back to work.

GATHER YOUR THOUGHTS

As we have tried to point out all through this book, only 5% of applicants get accepted each year. Is it the top 5% who get in? Hardly. No system is perfect, and some poorly qualified applicants are likely to slip through the cracks and be accepted. Many of these people will also fail along the way. This is inevitable, but some schools have a higher attrition rate than others. Take comfort in knowing you're not alone and you will get another chance.

In any case, **keep a positive attitude.** You will be a much stronger, and wiser, candidate next year. You will improve your grades, gain more experience, have a better understanding of the profession, and have more time to write a great essay.

DEVELOP A PLAN

Once you become ready to pick yourself up by the bootstraps, contact the schools that you applied to this year and ask for feedback on your application. This is a critical step, as you need to find out specifically where you are lacking as a candidate. Admissions committee members usually write down notes about your application or interview. Ask for specific areas that you need to improve in based on these comments. Generally, the comments will be relevant to experience, grades, understanding of the profession, poor essay, poor interview, or "weird behavior." The last may be hard to illicit from the program director or whomever may be giving you the feedback. Make a note of any suggestions and thank the committee for considering your application or for the interview. It is important to do this right away while your application is still fresh in their minds.

Once you accomplish the above, you are ready to return to chapter one and rewrite your goals. I hope by now you realize the value of doing this. Compile a concise plan of action to strengthen your application for next year. Do you need to take more classes? Do you need to take any classes over? Do you need more hands-on experience? How about your narrative—is it persuasive and motivating? Think carefully about how you can present yourself in a better light next year.

IMPLEMENT THE PLAN

Just do it! After you have a complete list of goals, begin working on them in their order of importance. For instance, if the program director told you that the committee is concerned with your ability to handle a rigorous science course load, enroll in some hard science courses at your local college next semester. Be sure to do well in these classes. If you are lacking experience, go out and start volunteering in the local emergency room. As a volunteer, you are usually considered an "insider" by the hospital and you may have a good shot at a paid job if one arises. Or, better yet, take a short course to become a certified nurse assistant (CNA) and get a paid job in a hospital or clinic. Jobs usually abound in this field.

Remember, the committee will look to see what you have done to improve your application over the past year. Too many people apply over and over again, but fail to make any positive changes.

NARRATIVE STATEMENT

When you fill out your application next year, be sure to write a brand new narrative statement, and obtain fresh letters of recommendation. This is very important. Let the committee know exactly what you have done to improve and strengthen your application. Point out that you followed their advice and took an extra class or gained more hands-on experience.

The purpose of writing a letter of recommendation is to provide the admissions committee with a detailed description of an applicant's abilities, rather than merely checking off a few boxes on a standard form. Too many applicants feel that as long as the letter is written by a so-called "big shot," the content is irrelevant. This is simply not true, and may hinder rather than help your application.

Let's look at a sample letter of recommendation for a candidate applying to PA school. Afterwards, we will dissect it and point out the three key elements that make up a great letter of reference.

Dear Ms. Dean:

Please accept this letter as a strong recommendation for John Smith's application as a student in your Physician Assistant Program. I am the current Dean of the College of Health and Human Performance at Mankato State University, and John was my student for four years and my teaching assistant for two years.

As a student, John was easily in the top ten percent of his peers for four years in a row. As a teaching assistant, he was rated the highest by over 122 students who have taken my classes. All students respected him and admired his presentations and leadership. He proved himself a dedicated, hard-working, and diligent young man.

John served for four years in the U.S. Navy as a corpsman, and his experience in that position would give great strength to his career as a Physician Assistant. He also spent time as an officer in the U.S. Air Force which explains his admirable ability to pay strict attention to detail.

This young man has a social conscience, high energy, a cooperative style, and has the uncanny ability to analyze complex problems in the health field in simple yet constructive context. His social graces are beyond reproach. John would make an outstanding PA. He really cares for people, and people care for him.

I strongly recommend John Smith for your Physician Assistant program.

Sincerely,

Robert R. Rockingham, Dr. P.H.
Dean, College of Health and Human Performance
Mankato State University

CONTENT

This letter contains the three key elements of an appropriate letter of reference:

1. Introduction and background of the writer.
2. Writer's relationship to the candidate.
3. Quantified claims versus general statements.

The purpose of the writer's introducing him/herself in the opening paragraph is to qualify as a legitimate reference. It shows that the reference truly knows the applicant and can honestly and objectively comment on his/her academic achievements, interpersonal and organizational skills, compassion, etc.

The writer should state his/her relationship to the candidate in order to offer an "expert" opinion. The writer should also state how long he/she has known the candidate and mention the circumstances that connect them.

Finally, quantify your claims. When we read applications, many people appear as though they can "walk on water." If the writer uses "meaningful specifics" versus "wandering generalities," he/she lends more credence to the letter.

Example: ". . . was rated the highest by over 122 students."

ID CANDIDATE'S STRENGTHS

A good recommendation letter does not simply recite the obvious: i.e., "Sue has a great GPA." It's quite obvious to the committee that Sue has a 3.7 GPA; we have her transcripts.

The writer should be more creative and spend enough time on the letter to make you stand out from the crowd. Again, be specific.

The writer is usually asked to evaluate you in several areas:

1. Academic performance
2. Interpersonal skills
3. Maturity
4. Adaptability/flexibility
5. Motivation for a career as a PA

The writer may comment on all of these areas or just a couple. In the area that he/she does comment on, however, the statements should be specific and relevant to the category selected.

For instance:

Academic performance: ". . . top ten percent of his peers."

Interpersonal skills: "He cares for people, and people care for him."

Maturity: "All students respected him and admired his presentations and leadership."

Adaptability/flexibility: ". . . has the uncanny ability to analyze complex problems . . . in simple yet constructive terms."

WHAT ABOUT WEAKNESSES?

We all have faults; the trick here is to have the evaluator mention a minor weakness and present it as though it is actually a strength. Mentioning a weakness lends objectivity and credibility to the letter of recommendation.

"John's strict attention to detail, at times, appeared to keep him late in the office. However, it is for this very reason that I believe he will make an excellent clinician, and will not miss any details when it comes to taking care of his patients."

ONE FINAL TIP

The writer should keep in mind that the reader of your application may have read a hundred others before yours. It's very important to keep the letters short, concise, specific, and personal. Be sure that the writer is recommending you for PA school and not "medical school." Also, be sure that the writer changes the name of the school with each application you send in.

I strongly recommend that you use the services of :

Universal Recommendations
P.O. Box 18700
Salt Lake City, UT 84118-0700
(801) 969-6085

Fill out the following sheet and keep a copy on your person at all times. Read this sheet every morning when you arise and every evening before you retire. By reading your goals daily, your subconscious mind will automatically begin working on helping you achieve them. This is a powerful technique, and it works!

My goal is to apply to the _____ PA program(s) and be accepted by _____ . **(Call each program that you will apply to and find out when candidates are notified about acceptance.)**

In order to achieve this goal, I will have to overcome the following obstacles: **(List all of the obstacles that you are likely to encounter: financial, relocation, convincing a spouse, etc.)**

_____
_____
_____
_____

The following people and organizations will help me achieve this goal: **(List everyone who can help you along the way; i.e., other PAs, the AAPA, your state chapter of the AAPA, friends, relatives, and us!)**

_____
_____
_____
_____

To be a competitive candidate I will have to: **(What will it take for you to stand out from the crowd? For example, will you have to take more science courses, gain more experience, work on getting a great letter of reference?)**

_____
_____
_____
_____

Beginning tonight, I will start putting into action the following plan: **(Ask yourself what you can do right now to get started.)**

_____
_____
_____
_____

The benefits I will receive from achieving this goal of **Getting into the PA school of my choice** include: **(Ask yourself, "What's in it for me? Why do I want to pursue this goal in the first place?"**

_____
_____
_____
_____

The following is a list of sample synonyms which will help you add more life and power to your essays. We encourage you to purchase a book of synonyms and refer to it frequently.

Articulate: crystal-clear, distinct, intelligible, eloquent, fluent, coherent

Logic: sound judgment, presence of mind, foresight, wisdom

Perceptive: sensitive, responsive, open, discriminating, insightful, quick, keen

Enthusiasm: intensity, fervor, glow, fire, zeal, passion, spirit, vivacity, emotion

Commitment: vow, assurance, obligation, guarantee, determination, promise

Practical: wise, tough, judicious, prudent, shrewd, canny, sharp, astute, clever

Crusader: fighter, visionary, advocate, champion, zealot, progressive

Realistic: practical, pragmatic, common-sense, down-to-earth, sensible, rational

Dependent: supported by, conditional, accessory to

Tactful: diplomatic, prudent, discreet, sensitive, clever, skillful, polished

Sincere: open, straight, earnest, fervent, dedicated, resolute, unpretentious

Poised: composed, calm, cool, mannered, polished, suave, unflappable

Integrity: honesty, veracity, candidness, honor

Teamwork: collaboration, interaction, cooperation, synergy, harmony, concert

Mature: refined, polished, self-sufficient, responsible, dependable, prudent

Flexible: adaptable, conformable, adjustable, malleable, compliant

Society of Air Force PAs
Box 6064
Sheppard AFB, TX 76311
(210) 221-7812

Society of Army PAs
6762 Candlewood Dr.
Fort Meyers, FL 33919-6402
(941) 482-2162

Alabama Society of PAs
PO Box 550274
Birmingham, AL 35255-0274
(205) 408-9497

Alaska Academy of PAs
PO Box 82684
Fairbanks, AK 99708
(907) 456-7687

Arizona State Assoc. of PAs
810 W. Bethany Home Rd.
Phoenix, AZ 85013
(602) 582-1246

Arkansas Academy of PAs
PO Box 218
Sparkman, AR 71763-0218
(501) 836-8101

California Academy of PAs
9778 Katella Ave. #115
Anaheim, CA 92804
(714) 539-1430

Colorado Academy of PAs
PO Box 4834
Englewood, CO 80155
(303) 770-6048

Connecticut Academy of PAs
PO Box 66
Bantam, CT 06750
(800) 493-9200

Delaware Academy of PAs
PO Box 25448
Wilmington, DE 19899
(302) 737-5768

D.C. Academy of PAs
800 K St., NW—Techworld Station
PO Box 50608
Washington, DC 20001
(301) 925-0119

Florida Academy of PAs
222 S. Westmonte Dr., #101
PO Box 150127
Altamonte Springs, FL 32715-0127
(407) 774-7880

Georgia Association of PAs
5300 Memorial Dr., #116
Stone Mountain, GA 30083
(404) 508-1482

Guahan Association of PAs
PO Box 6578
Tamuning, GU 96911
(671) 646-5825

Hawaii Academy of PAs
PO Box 30355
Honolulu, HI 96820
(808) 671-4713

Idaho Academy of PAs
777 N. Raymond, Suite 100 PA
Boise, ID 83704
(208) 344-7888

Illinois Academy of PAs
414 Plaza Dr., #209
Westmont, IL 60559
(217) 528-5230

Indiana Academy of PAs
101 W. Ohio Street, Suite 1414
Indianapolis, IN 46204
(888) 441-0423

Iowa PA Society
3200 Grand Ave.
Des Moines, IA 50312
(800) 441-2692

Kansas Academy of PAs
PO Box 20401
Wichita, KS 67208
(316) 681-7721

Kentucky Academy of PAs
PO Box 23251
Lexington, KY 40523-3251
(502) 441-4430

Louisiana Academy of PAs
3701 Division St., Suite 225
Metairie, LA 70002
(504) 922-4630

Downeast Association of PAs
RR 1, Box 1121A
Readfield, ME 04355
(207) 685-5531

Maryland Academy of PAs
PO Box 20277
Baltimore, MD 21284
(410) 625-1247

Massachusetts Association of PAs
PO Box 81362
Wellesley Hills, MA 02181-0004
(617) 893-4610, ext. 1350

Michigan Academy of PAs
2410 Woodlake Dr., Suite 440
Okemos, MI 48864
(517) 347-3398

Minnesota Academy of PAs
3433 Broadway St., NE, Suite 300
Minneapolis, MN 55413-1761
(612) 378-1875

Mississippi Academy of PAs
PO Box 5128
Biloxi, MS 39534
(601) 388-5541, ext. 5246

Missouri Academy of PAs
c/o 120 W. 16th St.
Mountain Grove, MO 65711
(417) 638-4045

Montana Academy of PAs
PO Box 35500-200
Billings, MT 59107
(406) 782-2195

Naval Association of PAs
Naval Hospital
PO Box 205
Corpus Christi, TX 78419
(800) 441-1173

Nebraska Academy of PAs
PO Box 31280
Omaha, NE 68131-0280
(402) 393-1415

Nevada Academy of PAs
PO Box 28877
Las Vegas, NV 89126
(702) 243-8500

New Hampshire Society of PAs
26 S. Main St., #166
Concord, NH 03301
(603) 622-6484

New Jersey State Society of PAs
PO Box 1282
Piscataway, NJ 08855-1282
(732) 235-4444

New Mexico Academy of PAs
7770 Jefferson NE, Suite 400
Albuquerque, NM 87109
(505) 768-5450

New York State Society of PAs
322 8th Ave., 14th Floor
New York, NY 10001-8001
(212) 206-8300

North Carolina Academy of PAs
1821 Hillandale Rd, Suite 1b-297
Durham, NC 27705
(800) 352-2271

North Dakota Academy of PAs
1809 Country West Rd.
Bismarck, ND 58501
(701) 858-3848

Ohio Association of PAs
700 Ackerman Rd., Suite 600
Columbus, OH 43202
(216) 256-4212

Oklahoma Academy of PAs
PO Box 53164
Oklahoma City, OK 73106
(405) 271-2058

Oregon Society of PAs
PO Box 20666
Keizer, OR 97307-0666
(503) 393-4899

Pennsylvania Society of PAs
PO Box 128
Greensburg, PA 15601
(412) 836-6411

Public Health Service Academy of
PAs
PO Box 16170
Phoenix, AZ 85011-6170
(800) 441-3716

Rhode Island Association of PAs
PO Box 5
Lincoln, RI 02865
(401) 331-3207

South Carolina Academy of PAs
100 Lexington Pointe Dr.
Columbia, SC 29223
(888) 442-0422

South Dakota Academy of PAs
1400 W. 22nd St.
Sioux Falls, SD 57105-1570
(605) 357-1518

Tennessee Academy of PAs
602 Gallatin Rd.
Oak Ridge, TN 37206
(615) 228-8695

Texas Academy of PAs
PO Box 80075
Austin, TX 78727-0075
(512) 370-1534

Utah Academy of PAs
50 North Medical Dr.
Bldg #528
Salt Lake City, UT 84132
(801) 567-6840

PA Academy of Vermont
c/o 591A Parker Hill Rd.
Springfield, VT 05156
(603) 543-3463

Veteran Affairs PA Association
PO Box 1109
330 East Lakeside St.
Madison, WI 53701
(800) 762-8977

Virginia Academy of PAs
11130 Main St., Suite #305
Fairfax, VA 22030
(703) 691-8515

Washington Academy of PAs
2033 Sixth Ave., Suite #1100
Seattle, WA 98121
(206) 726-2675

West Virginia Association of PAs
1527 Saxman Ave.
Morgantown, WV 26505
(800) 441-3544

Wisconsin Academy of PAs
PO Box 1109
330 East Lakeside St.
Madison, WI 53701-1109
(800) 762-8965

Wyoming Association of PAs
c/o Jane Cassel, PA-C
1522 East A St.
Casper, WY 82601
(307) 746-3582

ALABAMA

University of Alabama at
Birmingham-C,B
Surgeons Assistant Program
School of Health Related
Professions 222B
1714 Ninth Ave. South
Birmingham, AL 35294-1270

** University of South
Alabama-M
College of Allied Health Professions
Department of Physician Assistant
Studies
1504 Springhill Ave.
Room 4410
Mobile, AL 33604-3641
(334) 434-3641

CALIFORNIA

Charles R. Drew University
School of Medicine and Science-
C,B
Physician Assistant Program
College of Allied Health
1621 East 120th St.
Los Angeles, CA 90033
(213) 563-5879

University of Southern California-B
Primary Care Physician
Assistant Program
School of Medicine
1975 Zonal Ave., KAM B29
Los Angeles, CA 90033
(213) 342-1328

College of Osteopathic Medicine
of the Pacific-C
Physician Assistant Program
College Plaza
309 East Second St.
Pomona, CA 91766-1889
(909) 469-5378

University of California-Davis
Medical Ctr-C
Physician Assistant Program
Department of Family Practice
2525 Stockton Blvd.
Sacramento, CA 95817
(916) 734-3550

Stanford University/ Foothill
College-A,C
Primary Care Associate Program
School of Medicine
703 Welch Rd., Suite F-1
Palo Alto, CA 94304-1760
(415) 723-7043

COLORADO

University of Colorado-C,B,M
Child Health Associate/Physician
Assistant Program
School of Medicine
Box C-219
4200 East Ninth Ave.
Denver, CO 80262
(303) 270-4614

CONNECTICUT

Yale University School of
Medicine-GC
Physician Associate Program
47 College St., Suite 220
New Haven, CT 06510
(203) 785-4252

Quinnipiac College-GC,M
Physician Associate Program
275 Mount Carmel Ave.
Hamden, CT 06518-1908
(203) 281-8704

DISTRICT OF COLUMBIA

George Washington University-C,M
Physician Assistant Program
Himmelfarb 307
2300 Eye St., NW
Washington, DC 20037
(202) 994-2807

Howard University-B
Physician Assistant Program
College of Allied Health
6th & Bryant St., NW
Washington, DC 20059
(202) 806-7536

FLORIDA

University of Florida-M
Physician Assistant Program
College of Medicine
PO Box 100176
Gainesville, FL 32610-0176
(352) 395-7955

Nova Southeastern University-C,B
Physician Assistant Program
1750 NE 167th St.
North Miami Beach, FL 33162-3017
(305) 949-4000 ext. 1210

GEORGIA

Emory University School of
Medicine -M
Physician Assistant Program
1462 Clifton Rd., NE
Suite 280
Atlanta, GA 30322
(404) 727-7825

Medical College of Georgia-B
Physician Assistant Program
AE 1032
Augusta, GA 30322
(706) 721-2725

ILLINOIS

Cook County Hospital/Malcolm X
College-C,A
Physician Assistant Program
1900 West Polk St.
CCSN 801
Chicago, IL 60612
(312) 633-8029

Midwestern University-B,M
Physician Assistant Program
555 West 31st St.
Downers Grove, IL 60515
(312) 515-6171

Finch University of Health
Sciences/The Chicago Medical
School-M
3333 Green Bay Rd.
North Chicago, IL 60064-3095
(708) 578-3312

INDIANA

Butler University/Methodist
Hospital-B
Physician Assistant Program
College of Pharmacy & Health
Sciences
4600 Sunset Ave.
Indianapolis, IN 46208
(317) 940-9471

IOWA

University of Iowa-C,M
Physician Assistant Program
College of Medicine
2333 Steindler Bldg.
Iowa City, IA 52242
(319) 335-8922

University of Osteopathic
Medicine & Health Sciences-C,B
Physician Assistant Program
3200 Grand Ave.
Des Moines, IA 50312
(515) 271-1603

KANSAS

Wichita State University-B
Physician Assistant Program
College of Health Professions
Campus Box 43
Wichita, KS 67260
(316) 689-3011

KENTUCKY

University of Kentucky-C,B
Physician Assistant Program
A.B. Chandler Medical Center
Annex 2, Room 113
Lexington, KY 40536-0080
(606) 323-5743

LOUISIANA

Louisiana State University
Medical Center-B
Physician Assistant Program
School of Allied Health Professions
1501 Kings Highway
Shreveport, LA 71130
(318) 675-7317

MAINE

** The University of New
England-M
Physician Assistant Program
Hills Beach Rd.
Biddeford, ME 04005
(207) 283-0171 ext 2847

MARYLAND

Essex Community College-C
Physician Assistant Program
7201 Rossville Blvd.
Baltimore, MD 21237
(410) 780-6579

MASSACHUSETTS

Northeastern University-C,M*
Physician Assistant Program
202 Robinson Hall
Boston, MA 02115
(617) 373-3195

Springfield College/Baystate
Health Systems-C,B
Physician Assistant Program
263 Alden St.
Springfield, MA 01109
(748) 413-3136

MICHIGAN

University of Detroit Mercy-M
Physician Assistant Program
8200 West Outer Drive
PO Box 19900
Detroit, MI 48219-0900
(313) 993-6177

Western Michigan University-C,B
Physician Assistant Program
Kalamazoo, MI 49008-5138
(616) 387-5314

**Wayne State University-M
Physician Assistant Program
College of Pharmacy and Allied
Health
428 Shapero Hall
Detroit, MI 48202
(313) 577-1368

** Central Michigan University-M
Physician Assistant Program
205 Foust Hall
Mount Pleasant, MI 48859

MISSOURI

Saint Louis University-C,B
School of Allied Health
Professions
1504 South Grand Blvd.
St. Louis, MO 63104
(314) 577-8521

MONTANA

** Rocky Mountain College-B
Physician Assistant Program
1511 Polly Dr.
Billings, MT 59102
(406) 657-1190

NEBRASKA

University of Nebraska Medical
Center-C,M
Physician Assistant Program
600 South 42nd St.
Box 984300
Omaha, NE 68198-4300
(402) 559-5266

NEW JERSEY

University of Medicine and
Dentistry of New Jersey-C,M
Physician Assistant Program
Robert Wood Johnson Medical
School
675 Hoes Lane
Piscataway, NJ 08854
(908) 235-4444

NEW YORK

Albany–Hudson Valley-C,A
Physician Assistant Program
Albany Medical College
47 New Scotland Ave.
Albany, NY 12208
(518) 262-5251

The Brooklyn Hospital
Center/Long Island University-B
Physician Assistant Program
1 University Plaza
Brooklyn, NY 11201
(718) 488-1011

Touro College-B
Physician Assistant Program
School of Health Sciences
135 Carmen Rd., Bldg. 14
Dix Hills, NY 11746
(516) 673-3200 ext. 255

CUNY/Harlem Hospital Center-C,B
Physician Assistant Program
506 Lenox Ave.
WP-Room 619
New York, NY 10037
(212) 939-2525

Cornell University Medical College
Physician Assistant Program
"A Surgical Focus"
1300 York Ave.
Room F-1906
New York, NY 10021
(212) 746-5133/5134

Bayley Seton Hospital-C,B*
Physician Assistant Program
75 Vanderbilt Ave.
Staten Island, NY 10304
(781) 390-5570

State University of New York at
Stonybrook-C,B
Physician Assistant Program
School of Health Tech & Mgmt
#L2-052
Stony Brook, NY 11794-8202
(516) 444-3190

State University of New York at
Brooklyn-B
Health Science Center
450 Clarkson Ave., Box 1222
Brooklyn, NY 11203
(718) 270-2324

D'Youville College-B
Physician Assistant Program
320 Porter Ave.
Buffalo, NY 14201
(716) 881-7600

Rochester Institute of Technology-B
Physician Assistant Program
Department of Allied Health
85 Lomb Memorial Dr
Rochester, NY 14623-5603

Catholic Medical Center of
Brooklyn and Queens-C,B*
Physician Assistant Education
Program
89-15 Woodhaven Blvd.
Woodhaven, NY 11421
(718) 805-7599

Bronx Lebanon Hospital
Center-B
Physician Assistant Program
1650 Selwyn Ave., Suite 11D
Bronx, NY 10457
(718) 960-1255

**Wagner College/ Staten
Island University Hospital-B
Physician Assistant Program
74 Melville St.
Staten Island, NY 10309
(718) 390-3412

**Lemoyne College-C,B
Physician Assistant Program
Syracuse, NY 13214
(315) 445-4144

NORTH CAROLINA

Duke University
Medical Center-C,M
Physician Assistant Program
Box CFM-2914
Durham, NC 27710
(919) 286-8234

Bowman Gray School of Medicine
of Wake Forest University-C
Physician Assistant Program
1990 Beach St.
Winston-Salem, NC 27103
(910) 716-4356

** Methodist College
Physician Assistant Program
5400 Ramey St.
Fayetteville, NC 28311
(910) 630-7495

NORTH DAKOTA

University of North Dakota
School of Medicine-C
Physician Assistant Program
Health Sciences
501 North Columbia Rd.
PO Box 9037
Grand Forks, ND 58202-9037
(701) 777-2344

OHIO

Kettering College of Medical Arts-A
Physician Assistant Program
3737 Southern Blvd.
Kettering, OH 45429
(513) 296-7874

Cuyahoga Community College
(2 programs)-A
Physician Assistant Program
Surgeons Assistant Program
11000 Pleasant Valley Rd.
Parma, OH 44130
(216) 987-5363

OKLAHOMA

University of Oklahoma-M
Physician Associate Program
Health Sciences Center
PO Box 26901
Oklahoma City, OK 73190
(405) 271-2047
(405) 271-2058

PENNSYLVANIA

Gannon University-B
Physician Assistant Program
University Square
Erie, PA 16541
(800) 426-6668

Saint Francis College-C,B,M*
Department of Physician
Assistant Sciences
PO Box 600
Loretto, PA 15940-0600
(814) 472-3020

Medical College of Pennsylvania
and Hahnemann University-B,GC
Physician Assistant Program
School of Allied Health
Sciences and Humanities
Broad and Vine Streets
Mail Stop 504
Philadelphia, PA 19102-1192
(215) 762-7135

King's College-C,B
Physician Assistant Program
133 North River Street
Wilkes-Barre, PA 18711
(717) 826-5853

Duquesne University-C,M
Physician Assistant Program
John G. Ragos Sr.
School of Health Sciences
130 Health Sciences Bldg.
Pittsburgh, PA 15282
(412) 396-5000

** Beaver College
Physician Assistant Program
450 South Eaton Rd.
Glenside, PA 19038
(800) 776-2328

SOUTH CAROLINA

Medical University of South
Carolina-M
Physician Assistant Program
College of Health Professions
171 Ashley Ave.
Charleston, SC 29425-2703
(803) 792-2961

SOUTH DAKOTA

University of South Dakota-C,B
Physician Assistant Program
School of Medicine
414 East Clark Street
Vermillion, SD 57069-2390
(605) 677-5128

TENNESSEE

Trevecca Nazarene University-C,B
Physician Assistant Program
333 Murfreesboro Rd.
Nashville, TN 37210-2877
(615) 248-1225

TEXAS

University of Texas
Southwestern Medical Center-C,B
Physician Assistant Program
6011 Harry Hines Blvd.
Dallas, TX 75235-9090
(214) 648-1700

The University of Texas Medical
Branch-C,B
Physician Assistant Program
School of Allied Health Services
301 University Blvd.
Galveston, TX 77555-1028
(409) 772-3046

Baylor College of Medicine-M
Physician Assistant Program
Department of Community
Medicine
One Baylor Plaza, Rm. 633E
Houston, TX 77030
(713) 798-4619

UTAH

University of Utah-C
Physician Assistant Program
School of Medicine
50 North Medical Drive
Building 528
Salt Lake City, UT 84132
(801) 581-7764

WASHINGTON

University of Washington Medex
Northwest-C,B
Physician Assistant Program
4245 Roosevelt Way, NE
Seattle, WA 98105
(360) 548-2600

WEST VIRGINIA

The College of West Virginia-B
Physician Assistant Program
609 South Kanawah St.
Beckley, WV 25802
(304) 253-7351 ext 436

WISCONSIN

University of Wisconsin—Madison-
C,B
Physician Assistant Program
Room 1050 Medical Sciences
Center
1300 University Ave.
Madison, WI 53706
(608) 263-5620

UNIFORMED SERVICES

Interservice Physician Assistant
Program-C
HSHA-MM
Academy of Health Sciences
Fort Sam Houston, TX
78234-8765

Credentials Awarded
C   Certificate of Completion
A   Associate's Degree
B   Bachelor's Degree
B*   Bachelor's Degree Option
M   Master's Degree
M* Master's Degree Option
GC Graduate Certificate of
      Completion

** Physician Assistant programs which have provisional accreditation. Provisional accreditation is a time-limited accreditation status received by a new program that has not graduated a class. Applicants are encouraged to discuss with each program its accreditation status.

*Institutions with plans to apply for provisional accreditation:

Morally College
Riverside, CA

Ann Arundel Community College
Arnold, MD
(410) 541-2246

East Carolina University
Greenville, NC
(919) 328-4423

Union College
Lincoln, NE
(402) 486-2504

Medical College of Ohio
Toledo, OH
(419) 381-4172

Pacific University
Forest Grove, OR
(800) 933-9308

Pennsylvania College of
Technology
Williamsport, PA
(717) 326-3760

Allentown College
Center Valley, PA
(610) 282-4443

University of North Texas
Fort Worth, TX
(817) 735-2204

Alderson Broaddus College
Philippi, WV
(304) 457-1700

College of Health Sciences
Roanoke, VA
(540) 985-8563

** Operational and Unaccredited

Kirksville College of Osteopathic
Medicine
Phoenix, AZ
(800) 626-5266

Idaho State University
Pocatello, ID
(208) 236-4705

Lutheran College
Fort Wayne, IN
(319) 458-2451

Grand Valley State University
Allendale, MI
(616) 895-6611

Augsburg College
Minneapolis, MN
(612) 330-1039

Seton Hall University
Newark, NJ
(201) 982-5954

Daeman College
Amherst, NY
(716) 839-8551

Oregon Health Sciences University
Portland, OR
(503) 494-1484

Chatham College
Woodland Rd, PA
412-365-1405

Philadelphia College of Textiles
and Sciences
Philadelphia, PA
(215) 951-2800

University of Wisconsin at
LaCrosse
LaCrosse, WI
(608) 785-6620

Lock Haven University
Lock Haven, PA
(608) 893-2168

Interest has been expressed in establishing a PA program at the following institutions:

University of Alaska
Alaska

Red Rock Community College
Lakewood, CO

University of Hawaii
Hilo, HI

Southern Illinois University
School of Medicine
Carbondale, IL

Mankato State University
Mankato, MN

University of Montana
Missoula, MT

University of New Mexico
Albuquerque, NM

Seton Hill College
Greensburg, PA

University of Rhode Island
Providence, RI

Tennessee State University
with
Meharry Medical College
Nashville, TN

Eastern Virginia Medical School
Norfolk, VA

Medical College of Wisconsin in
Milwaukee
Milwaukee, WI

Marquette University
Marquette, WI

* Provisional accreditation is an accreditation status awarded to a new program (one that has not yet accepted students) and is time-limited.

** Operational and Unaccredited programs have students already and are going through the accreditation process.

APPLICANT PROFILE

Name:_____

Address:_____

Phone #:_____

Highest Degree at Application: Master's ____   Bachelor's ____
                                                  Assoc ____   Other ____

Colleges/Universities Attended

School #1

Dates: From _____   To: _____   School _____

Course of Study _____   Degree Earned _____

GPA _____

School #2

Dates: From _____   To: _____   School _____

Course of Study _____   Degree Earned _____

GPA _____

School #3

Dates: From _____   To: _____   School _____

Course of Study _____   Degree Earned _____

GPA _____

Please list your grades for the following courses:

Anatomy & Physiology I   _____

Anatomy & Physiology II   _____

Microbiology   _____

Chemistry I   _____

Chemistry II   _____

Organic Chem I   _____

Organic Chem II   _____

Psychology   _____

Please list all courses for which you receive a C, D, F, or W (withdrawal):

Please list all of your science grades (not already listed above):

Biology   _____

Chemistry   _____

Psychology   _____

Physics   _____

Medical Experience (Please list the indicated information for all medically related positions. Please list these in chronological order, beginning with the most recent, and specify each as volunteer (V) or paid (P) work. Calculate total, full-time months, using 40 hours/wk and 4 wks/month for your conversion. Use an additional sheet if necessary.

1._____ - _____   V or P   _____   _____
   (mos & yr)   (mos & yr)   circle one   position   (total mos)

   _____
   Description of Duties

   _____

2._____ - _____   V or P   _____   _____
   (mos & yr)   (mos & yr)   circle one   position   (total mos)

   _____
   Description of Duties

   _____

3._____ - _____   V or P   _____   _____
   (mos & yr)   (mos & yr)   circle one   position   (total mos)

   _____
   Description of Duties

   _____

4._____ - _____   V or P   _____   _____
   (mos & yr)   (mos & yr)   circle one   position   (total mos)

   _____
   Description of Duties

   _____

Based on the above information, we rank you a   1 2 3 4 5

1 = Definitely Interview
2 = Probably Interview
3 = Possibly Interview
4 = Probably Not Interview
5 = Definitely Not Interview

Our recommendations are as follows:

Please send us your suggestions or any personal stories regarding what was most effective in getting into the PA school of your choice. The preferred way to submit entries, suggestions, or corrections is via electronic mail, addressed to the authors:

Pasapg@iconn.net

You may also contact the publisher at:

Editorial Department
McGraw-Hill Medical Publishing Division
2 Penn Plaza, 12th Floor
New York, NY 10121

AJR Associates, visit our internet Website at:

www.Rodican.com

Otherwise, please send entries, neatly written or typed or on a disk (Microsoft Word), to First Aid for the USMLE Step 1, 720 Orange St. #2, New Haven, CT 06511–9046, Attention: Contributions. Please use the contribution and survey forms on the following pages. Each form constitutes an entry. (Attach additional pages as needed.)